Bone and Joint Infections

Editor

STEVEN K. SCHMITT

INFECTIOUS DISEASE CLINICS OF NORTH AMERICA

www.id.theclinics.com

Consulting Editor
HELEN W. BOUCHER

June 2017 • Volume 31 • Number 2

ELSEVIER

1600 John F. Kennedy Boulevard • Suite 1800 • Philadelphia, Pennsylvania, 19103-2899.

http://www.theclinics.com

INFECTIOUS DISEASE CLINICS OF NORTH AMERICA Volume 31, Number 2
June 2017 ISSN 0891–5520, ISBN-13: 978-0-323-53013-2

Editor: Kerry Holland
Developmental Editor: Donald Mumford

Infectious Disease Clinics of North America (ISSN 0891–5520) is published in March, June, September, and December by Elsevier Inc., 360 Park Avenue South, New York, NY 10010-1710. Periodicals postage paid at New York, NY and additional mailing offices. Subscription prices are $301.00 per year for US individuals, $588.00 per year for US institutions, $100.00 per year for US students, $357.00 per year for Canadian individuals, $734.00 per year for Canadian institutions, $428.00 per year for international individuals, $734.00 per year for international institutions, and $200.00 per year for Canadian and international students. To receive student rate, orders must be accompanied by name of affiliated institution, date of term, and the *signature* of program/ residency coordinator on institution letterhead. Orders will be billed at individual rate until proof of status is received. Foreign air speed delivery is included in all *Clinics* subscription prices. All prices are subject to change without notice. **POSTMASTER:** Send address changes to *Infectious Disease Clinics of North America,* Elsevier Health Sciences Division, Subcription Customer Service, 3251 Riverport Lane, Maryland Heights, MO 63043. **Customer Service: 1-800-654-2452 (US). From outside of the US and Canada, call 1-314-447-8871. Fax: 1-314-447-8029. E-mail: JournalsCustomerService-usa@elsevier.com (print support) or JournalsOnlineSupport-usa@elsevier.com (online support).**

Infectious Disease Clinics of North America is also published in Spanish by Editorial Inter-Médica, Junin 917, 1er A 1113, Buenos Aires, Argentina.

Reprints. For copies of 100 or more, of articles in this publication, please contact the Commercial Reprints Department, Elsevier Inc., 360 Park Avenue South, New York, New York 10010-1710. Tel. 212-633-3874, Fax: 212-633-3820, E-mail: reprints@elsevier.com

Infectious Disease Clinics of North America is covered in *MEDLINE/PubMed (Index Medicus), Current Contents/ Clinical Medicine, Science Citation Alert, SCISEARCH,* and *Research Alert.*

Contributors

CONSULTING EDITOR

HELEN W. BOUCHER, MD, FIDSA, FACP
Director, Infectious Diseases Fellowship Program, Division of Geographic Medicine and Infectious Diseases, Tufts Medical Center, Associate Professor of Medicine, Tufts University School of Medicine, Boston, Massachusetts

EDITOR

STEVEN K. SCHMITT, MD, FIDSA, FACP
Section Head, Section of Bone and Joint Infections, Department of Infectious Disease, Medicine Institute, Cleveland Clinic, Associate Professor, Cleveland Clinic Lerner College of Medicine, Cleveland, Ohio

AUTHORS

MAJA BABIC, MD
Assistant Professor of Medicine, Cleveland Clinic Lerner College of Medicine/Case Western Reserve University, Section of Bone and Joint Infections, Department of Infectious Disease, Cleveland Clinic, Cleveland, Ohio

ELIE F. BERBARI, MD
Professor of Medicine, Division of Infectious Diseases, Department of Internal Medicine, Mayo Clinic School of Medicine, Mayo Clinic, Rochester, Minnesota

BARRY D. BRAUSE, MD
Division of Infectious Diseases, Department of Medicine, Hospital for Special Surgery, Weill Cornell Medicine, New York, New York

IOANA CHIRCA, MD
Department of Infectious Diseases, University Hospital, Augusta, Georgia

ERIC O. GOMEZ-URENA, MD
Senior Associate Consultant, Division of Infectious Diseases, Department of Internal Medicine, Mayo Clinic, Rochester, Minnesota

MICHAEL W. HENRY, MD
Division of Infectious Diseases, Department of Medicine, Hospital for Special Surgery, Weill Cornell Medicine, New York, New York

JOHN I. HOGAN, MD
Clinical Fellow, Division of Infectious Diseases, Massachusetts General Hospital, Harvard Medical School, Boston, Massachusetts

ROCÍO M. HURTADO, MD, DTM & H
Associate Physician and Director, Mycobacterial Diseases Center, Division of Infectious Diseases, Massachusetts General Hospital, Assistant Professor, Harvard Medical School, Boston, Massachusetts

CAMELIA MARCULESCU, MD, MSCR
Associate Professor of Medicine, Division of Infectious Diseases, Medical University of South Carolina, Charleston, South Carolina

ANDY O. MILLER, MD
Division of Infectious Diseases, Department of Medicine, Hospital for Special Surgery, Weill Cornell Medicine, New York, New York

SANDRA B. NELSON, MD
Associate Physician and Director, Program in Musculoskeletal Infections, Division of Infectious Diseases, Massachusetts General Hospital, Assistant Professor, Harvard Medical School, Boston, Massachusetts

DOUGLAS R. OSMON, MD
Professor of Medicine, Division of Infectious Diseases, Department of Internal Medicine, Mayo Clinic School of Medicine, Mayo Clinic, Rochester, Minnesota

JOHN J. ROSS, MD, FIDSA
Department of Medicine, Brigham and Women's Hospital, Assistant Professor, Harvard Medical School, Boston, Massachusetts

STEVEN K. SCHMITT, MD, FIDSA, FACP
Section Head, Section of Bone and Joint Infections, Department of Infectious Disease, Medicine Institute, Cleveland Clinic, Associate Professor, Cleveland Clinic Lerner College of Medicine, Cleveland, Ohio

CLAUS S. SIMPFENDORFER, MD
Assistant Professor of Radiology, Cleveland Clinic Lerner College of Medicine/Case Western Reserve University, Section of Musculoskeletal Radiology, Imaging Institute, Cleveland Clinic, Cleveland, Ohio

AARON J. TANDE, MD
Assistant Professor of Medicine, Division of Infectious Diseases, Department of Internal Medicine, Mayo Clinic School of Medicine, Mayo Clinic, Rochester, Minnesota

THOMAS J. WALSH, MD
Division of Infectious Diseases, Department of Medicine, Hospital for Special Surgery; Departments of Pediatrics, Microbiology and Immunology, Weill Cornell Medicine, New York, New York

CHARALAMPOS G. ZALAVRAS, MD, PhD, FACS
Professor of Orthopaedics, Los Angeles County and University of Southern California Medical Center, Keck School of Medicine, University of Southern California, Los Angeles, California

Contents

Septic arthritis is a rheumatologic emergency that may lead to disability or death. Prompt evacuation of the joint, either by arthrocentesis at the bedside, open or arthroscopic drainage in the operating room, or imaging-guided drainage in the radiology suite, is mandatory. Methicillin-resistant *Staphylococcus aureus* (MRSA) has become a major cause of septic arthritis in the United States. MRSA joint infection seems to be associated with worse outcomes. Antibiotic courses of 3 to 4 weeks in duration are usually adequate for uncomplicated bacterial arthritis. Treatment duration should be extended to 6 weeks if there is imaging evidence of accompanying osteomyelitis.

Prosthetic joint infections (PJIs) are devastating complications after joint arthroplasty that continue to pose a diagnostic challenge. Currently, a single, stand-alone test with the adequate accuracy and reliability for diagnosis of PJI is not available; therefore, physicians who care for patients with PJI must rely on a combination of diagnostic tests for the diagnosis of PJI. This article reviews conventional laboratory test modalities, diagnostic accuracy and limitations of current tests, and novel emerging tests for the diagnosis of PJI.

Although uncommon, prosthetic joint infection is a devastating complication. This challenging condition requires a coordinated management approach to achieve good patient outcomes. This review details the general principles to consider when managing patients with prosthetic joint infection. The different medical/surgical treatment strategies and how to appropriately select a strategy are discussed. The data to support each strategy are presented, along with discussion of antimicrobial strategies in specific situations.

Total joint arthroplasty is a generally safe orthopedic procedure; however, infection is a potentially devastating complication. Multiple risk factors have been identified for development of prosthetic joint infections. Identification of patients at risk and preoperative correction of known risk factors, such as smoking, diabetes mellitus, anemia, malnutrition, and decolonization of *Staphylococcus* carriers, represent well-established actions to decrease the infection risk. Careful operative technique, proper draping and skin preparation, and appropriate selection and dosing of antimicrobials for perioperative prophylaxis are also very important in prevention of infection.

Reactive arthritis is classified as a spondyloarthropathy. Current concepts of disease suggest an infectious trigger, followed by inflammatory arthritis. Several mechanisms have been proposed to explain the interaction of host susceptibility and microorganism. Diagnosis relies on a compatible clinical syndrome and microbiologic confirmation of the pathogen. Antibiotic therapy seems useful in *Chlamydia*-triggered arthritis. The role of antibiotics in arthritis triggered by enteric pathogens is less clear. The role of tumor necrosis factor alpha inhibitors in therapy is evolving. Many patients have a course limited to a few months, but others experience extraarticular disease and more prolonged courses.

Pyogenic infections of the bony spinal column and the intervertebral discs are on a steady rise in an aging western population. Despite advanced medical imaging, this clinical entity of devastating consequences if missed, still presents a diagnostic conundrum and is plagued by an unacceptably long diagnostic delay. The aim of this article is to raise awareness of the heterogeneity of spinal infections paralleling the complex structure of the spinal column and neighboring soft tissues. Emphasis is placed on the clinical presentation and management of septic facet joints and psoas muscle abscesses associated with lumbar spondylodiscitis.

Imaging is often used to establish a diagnosis of musculoskeletal infections and evaluate the full extent and severity of disease. Imaging should always start with radiographs, which provide an important anatomic overview. MRI is the test of choice in most musculoskeletal infections because of its superior soft tissue contrast resolution and high sensitivity for pathologic edema. However, MRI is not always possible. Alternative imaging modalities including ultrasound scan, computed tomography, and radionuclide imaging may be used. This article reviews the individual imaging modalities and discusses how specific musculoskeletal infections should be approached from an imaging perspective.

Osteomyelitis is an ancient disease with varied pathophysiology. The several clinical syndromes associated with bone infection have specific clinical presentations and microbiology. Successful recognition and management of the disease requires a knowledge of these mechanisms and the organisms most common in each. Diagnosis is made by a combination of clinical examination, supportive blood testing, and appropriate radiography. With these elements in place, patient presentation can be placed in the framework of a staging system, which often helps to suggest the appropriate mix of antimicrobial and surgical therapies.

Open fractures are complex injuries that are associated with increased risk for complications, such as infection and nonunion. The goals of open fracture management are prevention of infection, fracture union, and restoration of function. These goals are best achieved by careful patient and injury assessment, early administration of systemic antibiotics supplemented by local delivery of antibiotics in severe injuries, thorough surgical debridement, wound management with soft tissue coverage if needed, and stable fracture fixation.

Fungi are rare but important causes of osteoarticular infections, and can be caused by a wide array of yeasts and molds. Symptoms are often subacute and mimic those of other more common causes of osteoarticular infection, which can lead to substantial delays in treatment. A high index of suspicion is required to establish the diagnosis. The severity of infection depends on the inherent pathogenicity of the fungi, the immune status of the host, the anatomic location of the infection, and whether the infection involves a foreign body. Treatment often involves a combination of surgical debridement and prolonged antifungal therapy.

Although less common as causes of musculoskeletal infection than pyogenic bacteria, both *Mycobacterium tuberculosis* and nontuberculous mycobacteria can infect bones and joints. Although tuberculous arthritis and osteomyelitis have been recognized for millennia, infections caused by nontuberculous mycobacteria are being identified more often, likely because of a more susceptible host population and improvements in diagnostic capabilities. Despite advances in modern medicine, mycobacterial infections of the musculoskeletal system remain particularly challenging to diagnose and manage. This article discusses clinical manifestations of musculoskeletal infections caused by *Mycobacterium tuberculosis* and nontuberculous mycobacteria. Pathogenesis, unique risk factors, and diagnostic and therapeutic approaches are reviewed.

INFECTIOUS DISEASE CLINICS OF NORTH AMERICA

RELATED INTEREST

Orthopedic Clinics, April 2017 (Vol. 48, Issue 2)
Infection
Frederick M. Azar, *Editor*

THE CLINICS ARE AVAILABLE ONLINE!
Access your subscription at:
www.theclinics.com

Preface

Musculoskeletal Infections: Meeting the Challenge

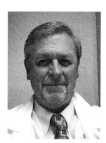

Steven K. Schmitt, MD, FIDSA, FACP
Editor

The field of musculoskeletal infections has continued to evolve in the interval since the last update on musculoskeletal infections appearing in the *Infectious Diseases Clinics of North America* in 2005. Despite pronouncements in the early 1980s that medical progress would turn the practitioners from multiple medical disciplines interested in infectious diseases into denizens of a fading field, quite the opposite has occurred. In a sense, it is precisely because of medical progress that the field of musculoskeletal infectious diseases has only increased in importance. Medical practice has extended lives with a dizzying array of therapies that leave patients immunocompromised by virtue of age, disease, or therapy. A variety of uncommon pathogens have emerged to affect bones and joints of patients with diminished immune systems. Even more common pathogens of native musculoskeletal tissue or hardware have been made difficult to treat by antimicrobial resistance born of both medical progress and gaps in antimicrobial stewardship. An exploding number of patients are recipients of orthopedic hardware, with an expectation of restoration of pain-free function. Unfortunately, a corresponding number of patients suffer the devastating consequences of infections of these devices, with limitation of device benefit, tremendous incremental expense, and loss of limb. Costing billions of dollars to treat and causing tremendous loss of function and productivity, musculoskeletal infections present a particular challenge to a health care system with tightened resources.

Fortunately, there has been increasing recognition of the value of cross-disciplinary interaction to advance our understanding of bone and joint infections. This issue offers a display of this, with topics encompassing infectious diseases, orthopedic surgery, rheumatology, and radiology. It is with a multidisciplinary focus that the topics and authors were selected. Ross leads a tour-de-force journey through septic arthritis of native joints. Gomez-Urena and colleagues offer practical insights to the often difficult task of diagnosing prosthetic joint infections; Tande and colleagues provide the latest in management recommendations, and Chirca and Marculescu review critical

Infect Dis Clin N Am 31 (2017) ix–x
http://dx.doi.org/10.1016/j.idc.2017.03.001
0891-5520/17/© 2017 Published by Elsevier Inc.

preventative strategies. Henry and colleagues discuss the latest in fungal musculo-skeletal infections, and Hogan and colleagues take on the difficult problem of myco-bacterial infections in orthopedics. There is increased understanding that certain pathogens trigger reactive spondyloarthropathy in susceptible patients; these are dis-cussed within this issue. In a like fashion, osteomyelitis, with its diverse pathogenesis and management issues, provides another critical area for infectious diseases focus. Babic and Simpfendorfer shine a light on the challenges of spine infection with atten-tion to less-discussed but nonetheless important variants, including facet joint infec-tions. Simpfendorfer gives the musculoskeletal radiologist's expert view of bone and joint infections. Zalavras provides an orthopedic surgeon's perspective on prevention of infection after trauma.

I would like to personally thank each of the authors, many of whom are colleagues in the Musculoskeletal Infection Society, and each of whom have exemplified a patient-centered approach to bone and joint infections. It is my hope as editor and the hope of the authors, who have pooled their many decades of combined, dedicated experience in the field, that readers will find here practical and engaging information to increase understanding of musculoskeletal infection and assist patients suffering with them.

Steven K. Schmitt, MD, FIDSA, FACP
Section of Bone and Joint Infections
Department of Infectious Disease, Medicine Institute
Cleveland Clinic
Cleveland Clinic Lerner College of Medicine
9500 Euclid Avenue
Desk G-21
Cleveland, OH 44195, USA

E-mail address:
schmits@ccf.org

Septic Arthritis of Native Joints

John J. Ross, MD

KEYWORDS

- Septic arthritis • Arthrocentesis • Synovial fluid • MRSA

KEY POINTS

- Septic arthritis is a true rheumatologic emergency that may lead to disability or death. Prompt evacuation of the joint, either by arthrocentesis at the bedside, open or arthroscopic drainage in the operating room, or imaging-guided drainage in the radiology suite, is mandatory.
- Arthrocentesis is diagnostic and therapeutic in patients with suspected septic arthritis. Patients should be treated empirically for septic arthritis if the synovial fluid white blood cell (WBC) count exceeds 50,000 cells/mm³. Patients with bacterial arthritis who are debilitated or immunosuppressed may have lower synovial fluid WBC counts.
- Methicillin-resistant *Staphylococcus aureus* (MRSA) is a major cause of septic arthritis in the United States; however, it is less prominent as a cause of septic arthritis in Europe. MRSA joint infection seems to be associated with worse outcomes. This may be due to its greater virulence, delays in initiation of appropriate antibiotics, and the older age of many affected patients.
- Antibiotic courses of 3 to 4 weeks in duration are generally adequate for uncomplicated bacterial arthritis. Treatment duration should be extended to 6 weeks if there is imaging evidence of accompanying osteomyelitis.

PATHOGENESIS

Septic arthritis of native (nonprosthetic) joints is uncommon but not rare, with approximately 2 cases per 100,000 people per year.[1] Occult bacteremia is probably the usual cause. Synovium is a vascular tissue that lacks a protective basement membrane, making it vulnerable to bacteremic seeding.[2] Minute breaks in the skin or mucous membranes may allow staphylococci and streptococci to gain access to the bloodstream. Gram-negative septic arthritis may arise from bacteremia from injection drug use or loss of integrity of the gastrointestinal or urinary tracts. Occasionally, septic arthritis is the direct result of penetrating trauma, such as human or animal bites or

The author has no disclosures.
Department of Medicine, Brigham and Women's Hospital, Harvard Medical School, 15 Francis Street, PBB-B420, Boston, MA 02115, USA
E-mail address: jross4@partners.org

Infect Dis Clin N Am 31 (2017) 203–218
http://dx.doi.org/10.1016/j.idc.2017.01.001
0891-5520/17/© 2017 Elsevier Inc. All rights reserved.

id.theclinics.com

errant injection drug use. This is the most common means of infection of the small joints of the hands and feet.[3] Rarely, bacterial arthritis may arise as a complication of arthroscopy or therapeutic joint injection with corticosteroids.

Most cases of septic arthritis are caused by gram-positive organisms. Enteric gram-negative rods account for 43% of community-acquired bacteremias, but cause only 10% of septic arthritis.[4,5] This likely relates to the superior ability of gram-positive organisms to bind connective tissue and extracellular matrix proteins. *Staphylococcus aureus*, the commonest cause of septic arthritis, produces several surface adhesins that bind to extracellular matrix proteins. Staphylococcal strains defective in microbial surface components recognizing adhesive matrix molecules are less arthritogenic in animal models.[6]

Joint damage in septic arthritis results from bacterial invasion, host inflammation, and tissue ischemia. Bacterial enzymes and toxins are directly injurious to cartilage. Cartilage may suffer "innocent bystander" damage, as host neutrophils release reactive oxygen species and lysosomal proteases. Cytokines activate host matrix metalloproteinases, leading to autodigestion of cartilage.[7] Ischemic injury also plays a role. Cartilage is avascular, and highly dependent on diffusion of oxygen and nutrients from the synovium. As purulent exudate accumulates, joint pressure increases, and synovial blood flow is tamponaded, resulting in cartilage anoxia.[8]

RISK FACTORS

The most robust risk factor for septic arthritis is preexisting joint disease (**Box 1**). Up to 47% of patients with bacterial arthritis have prior joint problems.[3] A high index of suspicion for septic arthritis should be maintained in patients with other rheumatologic conditions, such as rheumatoid arthritis (RA), osteoarthritis, gout, pseudogout, recent trauma, prior joint surgery, and systemic lupus erythematosus. Of these, RA is the most common, and is associated with worse outcomes.

Patients with RA are at high risk for bacterial arthritis from the combination of joint damage, immunosuppressive medications, and poor skin condition. Polyarticular

---

Box 1
Risk factors for septic arthritis of native joints

Preexisting joint diseases
   Rheumatoid arthritis
   Gout and pseudogout
   Osteoarthritis
   Lupus
   Trauma
   Recent surgery

Diabetes mellitus

Intravenous drug use

Cirrhosis

End-stage renal disease

Prednisone and other immunosuppressive medications

Skin diseases
   Psoriasis
   Eczema
   Skin ulcers

Human bite (fight bite)

disease and complications are common, functional outcomes are worse, and mortality is high in patients with RA with septic joints.[9] Diagnosis is often delayed because of the confusion of septic arthritis for a flare of RA.

In gouty patients with septic arthritis, inflammation results in shedding of synovial microtophi, obscuring the diagnosis. All patients with apparent gouty joints should also have routine Gram stain and culture performed to exclude concomitant septic arthritis.[10,11]

Two other broad categories of risk for septic arthritis are conditions causing loss of skin integrity, such as psoriasis, eczema, skin ulcers, and injection drug abuse, and conditions associated with compromised immunity, such as diabetes mellitus, renal failure, cirrhosis, and immunosuppressive drugs. Tumor necrosis factor blockers double the risk of septic arthritis in RA, and are associated with septic arthritis with intracellular pathogens, such as *Listeria* and *Salmonella*.[12] However, up to 22% of patients with septic arthritis have no medical risk factors and no underlying joint disease.[13]

A review of cases of septic arthritis from the National Hospital Discharge Survey revealed that the average age of patients with septic arthritis had risen from 37 years in 1979 to 51 in 2002. In recent years, patients had more comorbid medical conditions, had septic arthritis in the setting of complicated hospitalizations, and were more likely to have infection with antibiotic-resistant organisms. Overall in-hospital mortality was 2.6%, and was similar from 1979 to 2002.[14]

CLINICAL PRESENTATION

The diagnosis of septic arthritis is straightforward in the classic patient with fever, rigors, and a warm, swollen, and exquisitely painful joint. Unhappily, however, the clinical and laboratory diagnosis of septic arthritis is often imprecise. High-grade fever is present in only 58%,[13] although 90% have at least low-grade fever.[15] Serum leukocytosis is present in only 50% to 60% of patients.[13,15] Joint pain is blunted in the immunosuppressed, such as the RA patient on corticosteroids, leading to delayed diagnosis and more complications.[16]

Predictors of mortality in a multivariate analysis include age older than 65 years, confusion at presentation, and polyarticular disease. Predictors of joint damage include age older than 65 years, diabetes mellitus, and infection with β-hemolytic streptococci.[13]

JOINT DISTRIBUTION

The knee is the principal target of bacterial septic arthritis. Forty-five percent of septic arthritis cases in adults involve the knee.[3] Presumably, this is due to the imperfect human adaptation to bipedal locomotion. The enormous mechanical stresses about the knee joint particularly predispose it to injury.[17] Other large joints of the appendicular skeleton, including the hip (15%), ankle (9%), elbow (8%), wrist (6%), and shoulder (5%), are commonly involved in adults.[3] Polyarticular disease is seen in approximately 10% to 20% of cases. It is more common with gonococcal, pneumococcal, group B streptococcal, and gram-negative septic arthritis. Polyarticular septic arthritis is usually asymmetric, and involves an average of 4 joints. At least 1 knee is involved in 72% of cases. Major risk factors are steroid therapy, RA, lupus, and diabetes mellitus.[18]

SEPTIC ARTHRITIS OF CARTILAGINOUS JOINTS

Involvement of cartilaginous joints of the axial skeleton is infrequent, except in intravenous drug users.[19] Septic arthritis in intravenous drug users often affects the pubic symphysis and the sternoclavicular and sacroiliac joints. These joints are uncommonly infected in other patients with septic arthritis.[20–23]

The sacroiliac joint has a mobile synovial portion and an immobile fibrocartilaginous portion (syndesmosis). Sacroiliac septic arthritis is generally seen in younger patients, although cases in the elderly are sporadically observed. Patients present with buttock pain and fever. It may be difficult to localize the pain on examination. The FABERE test (Flexion, ABduction, External Rotation, and Extension) stresses the sacroiliac joint. It is performed on the supine patient by placing the ipsilateral medial malleolus on the opposite knee. The ipsilateral knee is depressed, with pressure exerted on the opposite superior iliac spine. Pain is elicited in sacroiliitis, although the FABERE test is not specific for infection.[20,21]

The pubic symphysis is a nonsynovial cartilaginous joint. Infection of the pubic symphysis presents with fever, suprapubic and hip pain, and a waddling, antalgic gait. Pubic symphysis septic arthritis is rare. Most cases occur in patients with well-defined risk factors, such as intravenous drug use, pelvic malignancy or surgery, and athletes, such as soccer players, who are prone to overuse injuries of the hip adductors and pubic periostitis.[22]

The sternoclavicular joint is a synovial joint, containing a fibrocartilaginous disc that separates it into 2 compartments. Infection of the sternoclavicular joint may account for up to 17% of septic arthritis in intravenous drug users. This joint is likely infected from phlebitis or valvulitis of the underlying subclavian vein, after injection of contaminated drugs into the upper extremity. Computed tomography (CT) or MRI should be obtained routinely in patients with sternoclavicular septic arthritis, given the high frequency of complications requiring surgery, such as chest wall abscess or mediastinitis.[23]

BACTERIOLOGY
Staphylococcus aureus

The most common cause of septic arthritis is *Staphylococcus aureus*, which accounts for 52% of cases (**Table 1**). Only 46% have an underlying focus of staphylococcal infection, such as cellulitis.[24] In the remainder, septic arthritis presumably arises as a consequence of transient bacteremia from a skin or mucous membrane source. Outcomes may be poor. Mortality ranges from 7% to 18%, and osteomyelitis or loss of joint function occurs in up to 27% to 46%.[13,15]

Methicillin-resistant *S aureus* (MRSA) is increasing in importance in septic arthritis, especially in the United States. In a recent series in Boston, 25% of septic arthritis cases were caused by MRSA.[25] All cases were associated with chronic illness, older age, and health care exposure. A high proportion of cases due to MRSA also has been seen in series from Detroit (21%) and northern California (50%).[26,27] MRSA caused 36% of septic arthritis in a recent series from São Paolo, Brazil, and 42% in a series from in Taiwan.[28,29] MRSA is less common as a cause of septic arthritis in Europe, causing 15% of cases in a French series, and only 5% of Swiss cases.[30,31]

β-hemolytic Streptococci

Group B streptococci (*Streptococcus agalactiae*) have emerged as invasive pathogens in the elderly, especially those with diabetes, cirrhosis, and neurologic disease.[32] At one center, group B streptococci increased from 1% of septic arthritis cases in the 1980s, to 6% in the 1990s.[33] In 2 other recent series, group B streptococci caused 10% of septic arthritis.[34,35] Bacteremia was seen in 66%, polyarticular disease in 32%, and mortality was 9%.[34] Other β-hemolytic streptococci, particularly group A

Table 1
Microbiology of 505 cases of septic arthritis in large series reporting data from 1999–2013

Bacteria	Number (%)
Staphylococci	282 (56)
Methicillin-sensitive *Staphylococcus aureus* (MSSA)	214 (42)
Methicillin-resistant *S aureus* (MRSA)	51 (10)
Coagulase-negative staphylococci	17 (3)
Streptococci	83 (16)
Unspecified streptococcal species	56 (11)
Viridans streptococci	7 (1)
Streptococcus pneumoniae	5 (1)
Other streptococcal species	15 (3)
Gram-negative rods	78 (15)
Pseudomonas aeruginosa	30 (6)
Escherichia coli	14 (3)
Proteus species	5 (1)
Klebsiella species	5 (1)
Others	21 (4)
Others	62 (12)
Polymicrobial	25 (5)
Anaerobes	3 (0.6)
Mycobacterium tuberculosis	9 (1.8)
Neisseria gonorrhoeae (gonococcus)	6 (1.2)
Miscellaneous	19 (4)

Data from Refs.[26,29–31]

streptococci (*Streptococcus pyogenes*), may cause an equally virulent form of septic arthritis in adults, although with lesser frequency.

Pneumococcus

Streptococcus pneumoniae caused 6% of cases of septic arthritis in an older literature review,[5] but it appears to be declining in importance as a cause of septic arthritis. In a more recent series, only 3% of septic arthritis was pneumococcal.[36] This may be attributable to increased herd immunity from childhood pneumococcal vaccination, which has been associated with fewer cases of invasive pneumococcal disease in adults.[37]

As with septic arthritis caused by group B streptococci, pneumococcal septic arthritis is notable for a high frequency of bacteremia and polyarticular disease. Only 50% have an underlying focus of pneumococcal disease, such as pneumonia. Mortality in adults is high (19%), although functional outcomes are good in 95% of survivors. Drug resistance may be an increasing problem.[5]

Gonococcal Arthritis

Neisseria gonorrhoeae, once the leading cause of septic arthritis in young adults in the United States, has dwindled in importance since the 1980s, and now accounts for only 1% of septic arthritis cases. However, recent increases in high-risk sexual behavior and rising rates of gonorrhea resistant to fluoroquinolones and azithromycin suggest that epidemic gonorrhea could be poised for a comeback.

Gonococcal septic arthritis is a distinct clinical syndrome, with a good prognosis. Seventy-five percent of cases occur in women; menses and pregnancy increase the risk of disseminated gonococcal infection[38]; 72% of cases are polyarticular.[24] Patients may experience a fleeting and migratory polyarthritis, or a more conventional septic arthritis picture of several hot, swollen, and exquisitely tender joints. Knee involvement is most common. The characteristic hemorrhagic pustules of disseminated gonococcal infection are found in 42% of patients, and tenosynovitis in 21%. Urinary signs or symptoms are present in only 32%. Gonococci are recovered from joint fluid in less than 50% of cases. This is probably largely because of the difficulty in recovering these fastidious organisms from cultures, but it may also indicate that some cases of gonococcal arthritis are immune-mediated.[38] Complete recovery is the rule with appropriate therapy, and sequelae are rare.

Enteric Gram-Negative Rods

Gram-negative rods cause approximately 10% to 15% of adult septic arthritis. Two major groups are at risk: elderly patients with comorbid medical conditions, and young intravenous drug users.[39,40] Outcomes are typically better in the latter group. Recent data suggest that outcome of gram-negative septic arthritis in older patients may be relatively good with prompt diagnosis and aggressive therapy, with mortality rates of only 5%, and poor functional outcomes in 32%. Perhaps surprisingly, an underlying source of gram-negative septic arthritis, such as a urinary tract infection, is found in only 50% of older patients.[41] Gram-negative bacilli have waned in importance as a cause of septic arthritis in injection drug users in recent years.

Meningococcal Arthritis

The incidence of arthritis in invasive meningococcal disease is as high as 14%. The usual presentation is a monoarthritis or oligoarthritis, involving the knee and other large joints. In most cases, arthritis develops several days into antibiotic therapy, and the joint fluid is sterile. Synovial fluid immune complexes have been detected in several of these patients, suggesting an immunologic basis of arthritis.[42,43] Less commonly, patients present with an isolated septic joint (primary meningococcal arthritis), or an arthritis-dermatitis syndrome akin to disseminated gonococcal infection.[44] Joint outcomes in meningococcal arthritis are usually excellent, with complete preservation of function.[42]

SEPTIC ARTHRITIS IN SPECIFIC POPULATIONS OR AFTER UNUSUAL EXPOSURES
Coagulase-Negative Staphylococci and Postarthroscopic Septic Arthritis

Most isolates of coagulase-negative staphylococci from native joints are contaminants, but they can be true joint pathogens after arthroscopy, anterior cruciate ligament reconstruction, and other orthopedic procedures. Septic arthritis after arthroscopy is associated with intra-articular corticosteroids, longer operating times, multiple prior procedures, and chrondroplasty or soft tissue debridement. Coagulase-negative staphylococcal joint infection tends to present in an indolent fashion, with low-grade fever, normal peripheral leukocyte counts, and mild to moderate joint symptomatology. Two weeks of parenteral antibiotics are usually curative for postarthroscopic septic arthritis.[45] Septic arthritis complicating anterior cruciate ligament reconstruction is treated with aggressive arthroscopic irrigation and debridement, followed by antibiotics for 6 weeks. Grafts usually can be retained, if they appear intact on arthroscopic inspection.[46]

Mycobacterium Tuberculosis

Tuberculosis causes up to 2% of septic arthritis. A high clinical suspicion is required to diagnose mycobacterial joint infection. Compared with typical septic arthritis, which presents with a hot and exquisitely painful joint, tuberculous arthritis usually pursues an indolent course. Patients often have gradually progressive joint pain and swelling that mimics osteoarthritis. Symptoms are often present for more than a year before diagnosis. Fever and weight loss are usually absent, and only 50% of patients have chest radiographs suggestive of tuberculous infection. Because delayed diagnosis is typical, abscesses, cutaneous fistulae, osteomyelitis, and joint deformities are often present. Synovial biopsy for histology and mycobacterial culture is the highest yield diagnostic procedure. Treatment of tuberculous arthritis is similar to that of tuberculosis at other sites. For drug-sensitive disease, regimens lasting 6 to 9 months are usually curative.[47]

Brucellosis

Brucella species are a common cause of subacute or chronic arthritis in countries in which livestock are not vaccinated and unpasteurized dairy products are consumed. In a recent Israeli series, 11% of septic arthritis was due to brucellosis, with most cases occurring in rural Arab populations.[48] In the United States, most cases are seen in immigrants from Latin America and the Middle East. The sacroiliac joint is involved in up to 54% of patients, for unclear reasons. Spondylitis occurs in 7%. Other patients present with monoarthritis or oligoarthritis, with lower extremity predominance. It has been suggested that brucellar arthritis may be reactive.[49] Brucellosis is diagnosed by blood culture or serology. The highest cure rates were reported with the combination of doxycycline for 45 days and streptomycin for 14 days.[50]

Foreign Body Synovitis and Plant Thorn Injuries

Penetrating joint injuries involving thorny plants, sea urchin spines, wood splinters, and other foreign bodies may cause a chronic synovitis. This arthritis is usually allergic in nature. The plant pathogen *Pantoea agglomerans*, however, has been implicated in several cases of thorn injuries.[51] There is also a report of *Nocardia asteroides* infection in this setting.[52] Thorn fragments and other synovial foreign bodies are best localized by ultrasound. Treatment is arthrotomy, with complete resection of foreign matter, and appropriate antibiotics based on joint cultures.

Human and Animal Bites

Human bites cause polymicrobial infection, involving aerobic bacteria, such as staphylococci; α- and β-hemolytic streptococci; oral gram-negative rods, such as *Eikenella corrodens*; and oral anaerobes, including *Prevotella*, *Fusobacterium*, and *Peptostreptococcus* species.[53] Animal bites have a similar bacteriology, with *Pasteurella multocida* as an important additional pathogen.[54,55] Treatment relies on drainage and debridement of devitalized tissues, careful assessment for tenosynovitis, and use of ampicillin-sulbactam, or a regimen with similar aerobic and anaerobic activity.

Whipple Disease

The multisystem disorder, Whipple disease, is caused by the fastidious actinomycete *Tropheryma whippelii*. In 63% of cases, a migratory, nondestructive, peripheral arthritis is the initial manifestation, preceding the onset of abdominal pain, diarrhea, malabsorption, and weight loss by a mean of 8 years in 1 series. Because patients often have HLA-B27 positivity, the arthritis may be mistakenly treated with immunosuppressive medication, precipitating gastrointestinal symptoms.[56,57] Fever, lymphadenopathy, hyperpigmentation, and cardiac and neurologic involvement also may be prominent. Diagnosis is usually made on the basis of small bowel biopsy, although polymerase chain reaction of synovial fluid also may be useful.[58] Two weeks of parenteral ceftriaxone is recommended as initial therapy, followed by oral trimethoprim-sulfamethoxazole for at least 1 year.[59]

Mycoplasmas and Ureaplasmas

True septic arthritis caused by mycoplasmas and ureaplasmas is unusual, occurring almost exclusively in the setting of hypogammaglobulinemia or organ transplantation. Diagnosis depends on polymerase chain reaction or cultivation on special media. Good outcomes have been reported with the combination of doxycycline and quinolones over weeks to months.[60–62]

Intravenous Drug Users

Before 1983, *Pseudomonas aeruginosa* caused 64% of reported septic arthritis in intravenous drug users, with *S aureus* responsible for only 10%. After 1983, the roles of these pathogens were reversed: *P aeruginosa* resulted in only 9% of septic arthritis in intravenous drug users, whereas *S aureus* caused 71%.[19] This switch is explained by shifting patterns of intravenous drug use. In 1983, in response to an epidemic of pentazocine abuse, the manufacturer coformulated it with the narcotic antagonist naloxone. With oral administration, naloxone is rapidly inactivated, but with injection, it negates the intoxicating effect of pentazocine. Thereafter, heroin supplanted pentazocine as the drug of choice among injection drug users.[63] Intravenous drug users often inject drugs with the most convenient water supply, such as puddles in alleys or toilet water. In one study, 81% of injection drug users reported injecting in public toilets in the past 6 months, and 80% in the street.[64] Unlike pentazocine, which dissolves in water at room temperature, heroin must be heated to dissolve, typically by boiling in a spoon held over a flame. This process of "cooking" reduces contamination with environmental bacteria, such as *Pseudomonas* sp. Cooking does not diminish the risk of staphylococcal infection, probably because the bacterial source is likely a colonized skin site, rather than environmental water.

Children

In pediatric septic arthritis, knee involvement is not as dominant as in adults. The knee and hip are infected in one-third of cases each in children.[65] Staphylococci and streptococci are responsible for most cases. *Haemophilus influenzae* type b septic arthritis is now uncommon because of the protection provided by conjugate vaccines.[66]

Kingella kingae, one of the fastidious gram-negative rods of the HACEK group, has recently been recognized as an important cause of septic arthritis, osteomyelitis, and intervertebral diskitis in children younger than 2 years. *Kingella* septic arthritis is often preceded by pharyngitis or stomatitis. Seasonality of infection has been observed, perhaps related to viral infection or other cofactors. There is 1 report of an outbreak of invasive *Kingella* infections in a day care. Routine inoculation of pediatric synovial fluid specimens into aerobic blood culture bottles has been recommended, instead of direct plating of specimens on solid media, to improve recovery of *Kingella*.[67–69]

Community-acquired MRSA is a major pediatric pathogen in the United States. In a recent series from Texas, MRSA caused 62% of pediatric musculoskeletal infection.[70] Disabling sequelae, such as decreased joint range of motion and limping gait, may be more common with MRSA infection.[71]

Prosthetic Joints

The diagnosis and management of prosthetic joint infection are reviewed elsewhere in this issue.

DIAGNOSIS: PROBLEMS AND PITFALLS

Gram stain and culture of synovial fluid should be sent in any case of undiagnosed arthritis. Antibiotic therapy ideally should be deferred until after synovial fluid is sampled. The involvement of rheumatology, orthopedic surgery, or interventional radiology may be necessary to obtain synovial fluid.

Gram stains of synovial fluid are helpful when positive, but they are not sensitive for the diagnosis of septic arthritis. Gram stains are positive in 71% of gram-positive septic arthritis,[15] 40% to 50% of cases of gram-negative septic arthritis,[39–41] and fewer than 25% of cases of gonococcal septic arthritis.[2]

Patients should be treated empirically for septic arthritis when synovial fluid white blood cell (WBC) counts exceed 50,000 cells/mm^3,[72] although gout and pseudogout also commonly cause WBC counts of this magnitude.[73] Unfortunately, lower WBC counts do not exclude septic arthritis. In one study, one-third of patients with septic arthritis had synovial fluid WBCs of fewer than 50,000 cells/mm^3,[35] and in another study, 50% of patients with septic arthritis had synovial fluid WBC counts fewer than 28,000 cells/mm^3.[74] Immunosuppressed patients may lack synovial leukocytosis altogether. Synovial chemistry tests, such as glucose and protein, are not useful in the diagnosis of septic arthritis.[75] Serum inflammatory markers, such as WBC counts, erythrocyte sedimentation rates, and C-reactive protein are also of limited value, as they are elevated in crystalline arthropathies and other conditions that may mimic septic arthritis.[76] However, the serum procalcitonin level shows some promise as a marker for septic arthritis.[77,78]

Blood cultures should be obtained in all patients with suspected septic arthritis. At least one-third of patients with septic arthritis have associated bacteremia. In up to 14% of patients, a bacteriologic diagnosis is made only on the basis of blood cultures.[1,24] Serologic testing for Lyme disease should be obtained from patients with undiagnosed inflammatory arthritis in endemic areas, particularly if Gram stain and culture of synovial fluid are negative.

The diagnosis of gonococcal septic arthritis may be elusive. Fewer than 50% of synovial fluid cultures are positive, even when appropriately subcultured onto chocolate agar. The diagnosis is usually based on a clinical syndrome compatible with disseminated gonococcal infection, and isolation of N gonorrhoeae from cultures or nucleic acid amplification tests from cervical, urethral, rectal, or oropharyngeal samples. Bacteremia is uncommon in disseminated gonococcal infection, despite the frequency of polyarticular involvement.[2,24,38]

Approximately 20% of cases of suspected septic arthritis have negative cultures of synovial fluid on solid media. There are many possible explanations for this phenomenon: the clinical diagnosis of septic arthritis may be mistaken; synovial fluid was obtained after the initiation of antibiotics; small numbers of bacteria were present, perhaps because of brisk neutrophil phagocytosis; the quantity of synovial fluid plated was inadequate; or infecting bacteria may have had fastidious growth requirements. Many of these problems may be overcome by inoculation of synovial fluid into blood culture bottles. Antibiotics and other bacterial inhibitors, such as complement, may be diluted in blood culture bottles; lytic agents present in most blood culture media, such as saponin, may release intracellular bacteria; larger amounts of synovial fluid can be inoculated into blood cultures; and blood cultures better support the growth of fussy organisms, such as *Kingella* and nutritionally variant streptococci. Several studies have shown a higher yield for pathogens, and fewer contaminants, with inoculation of synovial fluid into blood cultures, compared with solid media.[79–81]

CT or MRI may confirm the presence of effusions and inflammation in joints that are difficult to assess clinically, such as the shoulder, hip, sacroiliac, and sternoclavicular joints (**Fig. 1**). It may also help to exclude osteomyelitis in adjacent bones.

ANTIBIOTIC THERAPY

Because synovial fluid tests lack precision for diagnosing septic arthritis, the threshold for starting antibiotics should be low. Patient epidemiology may help tailor empiric therapy toward likely organisms. However, because septic arthritis is so rapidly destructive, broad-spectrum antibiotics are usually warranted until culture data are available. Given the increasing importance of MRSA as a cause of septic arthritis, initial antibiotic regimens should generally include an antibiotic active against MRSA, such as vancomycin. Cefazolin is a reasonable alternative in areas with a low prevalence of MRSA. A drug active against gram-negative bacilli, such as cefepime or an antipseudomonal beta-lactam, should be added if patients are critically ill or have a higher risk of gram-negative infection, such as the elderly, the immunocompromised, or intravenous drug users.

Septic arthritis associated with human or animal bites should be treated with agents active against oral flora, such as ampicillin-sulbactam. Sexually active patients with clinical syndromes suggestive of disseminated gonococcal infection should receive ceftriaxone. Recommendations for empiric antibiotic therapy of suspected septic arthritis are summarized in **Box 2**.

Once the causative organism has been identified, therapy should be narrowed based on sensitivity data. Data on duration of therapy are scanty. In general, septic arthritis in adults should be treated for at least 3 weeks, which may include a period of step-down oral therapy. In children with uncomplicated septic arthritis, as few as 10 days of antibiotic therapy may suffice.[82] Gonococcal septic arthritis can be treated with 2 weeks of ceftriaxone. Because osteomyelitis is common in infections of cartilaginous joints, such as the sternoclavicular and sacroiliac joints, antibiotic courses of 6 weeks are recommended.[23]

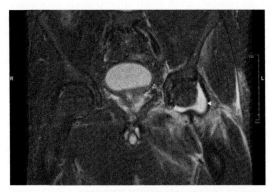

Fig. 1. A 35-year-old man with a history of intravenous drug use presented with a painful left hip. Pelvic MRI (coronal cut) showed a moderate effusion of the left hip joint (*arrow*), with diffuse edema involving nearly all of the muscles of the left hip. Blood cultures and synovial fluid cultures grew methicillin-sensitive *S aureus*.

Box 2
Empiric antibiotic therapy for suspected septic arthritis of native joints

Gram-positive cocci on Gram stain of synovial fluid
   High-prevalence area for methicillin-resistant *Staphylococcus aureus* (MRSA)
     Vancomycin 1 g intravenous (IV) every 12 hours
   Low-prevalence area for MRSA
     Cefazolin 2 g IV every 8 hours

Gram-negative cocci on Gram stain of synovial fluid, or clinical syndrome suggestive of
disseminated gonococcal infection
   Ceftriaxone 1 g IV every 24 hours PLUS
   Azithromycin 1 g orally (single dose)

Gram-negative rods on Gram stain of synovial fluid
   Cefepime 2 g IV every 8 hours or piperacillin-tazobactam 4.5 g IV every 6 hours

No organisms seen on Gram stain
   Vancomycin 1 g IV every 12 hours (cefazolin may be used in areas of low MRSA prevalence)
   In the elderly, immunocompromised, critically ill, or intravenous drug users, add an
   antipseudomonal beta-lactam, such as cefepime or piperacillin-tazobactam

---

Historical series of septic arthritis have shown that a large proportion of patients with suspected septic arthritis have negative joint fluid cultures. These patients have similar clinical and epidemiologic features compared with those with bacteriologically confirmed septic arthritis. It is reasonable to complete a short course of oral antibiotic therapy in these patients.[83]

JOINT DRAINAGE

In the preantibiotic era, some patients with septic arthritis had good outcomes with aggressive joint irrigation alone. Today, septic arthritis is managed with antibiotics combined with joint drainage by arthroscopy, arthrocentesis, or arthrotomy. Joint drainage decompresses the joint, improves blood flow, and removes bacteria, toxins, and proteases. Arthrocentesis should be repeated daily until effusions resolve and cultures are negative. There is general agreement that surgical drainage is indicated for septic arthritis of the hip, failure to respond after 5 to 7 days of antibiotics and arthrocentesis, and soft tissue extension of infection. The shoulder joint should be drained either surgically or under radiologic guidance.[84,85] Retrospective data suggest that patients with RA have better functional outcomes with surgical management.[9]

Patients with sternoclavicular septic arthritis often respond poorly to medical management, especially when antibiotic therapy is delayed. Thoracic surgery should be consulted in these patients to assess the need for sternoclavicular joint excision and pectoralis flap grafting.[86,87] Chest imaging with CT or MRI should be obtained routinely to exclude osteomyelitis, chest wall abscess, and mediastinitis.

No good data show a superiority of surgical drainage over arthrocentesis. In fact, one meta-analysis, and a more recent retrospective study, demonstrated better functional outcomes with arthrocentesis compared with surgery, although mortality was higher in patients treated with arthrocentesis.[13,88] Selection bias probably explains these differences. Critically ill patients are poor surgical candidates, whereas otherwise stable patients with severe septic arthritis are more likely to undergo surgical drainage. Randomized clinical trials of arthrocentesis compared with surgical or arthroscopic drainage are needed.

A recent study showed a significant benefit of dexamethasone therapy in preventing disability in children with septic arthritis, but no data exist to recommend its use in adults.[89]

Aggressive rehabilitation is essential to prevent joint contractures and muscle atrophy. Patients should be mobilized as soon as pain allows. Although early reviews recommended joint immobilization in the acute phase of infection,[2] in animal models of septic arthritis, more cartilage degeneration and adhesions were seen in immobilized animals, compared with animals treated with continuous passive motion devices.[90]

REFERENCES

1. Cooper C, Cawley MI. Bacterial arthritis in an English health district: a 10 year review. Ann Rheum Dis 1986;45:458–63.
2. Goldenberg DL, Reed JI. Bacterial arthritis. N Engl J Med 1985;312:764–71.
3. Kaandorp CJ, Dinant HJ, van de Laar MA, et al. Incidence and sources of native and prosthetic joint infection: a community based prospective survey. Ann Rheum Dis 1997;56:470–5.
4. Haug JB, Harthug S, Kalager T, et al. Bloodstream infections at a Norwegian university hospital, 1974–1979 and 1988–89: changing etiology, clinical features, and outcome. Clin Infect Dis 1994;19:246–56.
5. Ross JJ, Saltzman CL, Carling P, et al. Pneumococcal septic arthritis: review of 190 cases. Clin Infect Dis 2003;36:319–27.
6. Patti JM, Bremell T, Krajewska-Pietrasik D, et al. The *Staphylococcus aureus* collagen adhesin is a virulence determinant in experimental septic arthritis. Infect Immun 1994;62:152–61.
7. Shirtliff ME, Mader JT. Acute septic arthritis. Clin Microbiol Rev 2002;15:527–44.
8. Stevens CR, Williams RB, Farrell AJ, et al. Hypoxia and inflammatory synovitis: observations and speculation. Ann Rheum Dis 1991;50:124–32.
9. Gardner GC, Weisman MH. Pyarthrosis in patients with rheumatoid arthritis: a report of 13 cases and a review of the literature from the past 40 years. Am J Med 1990;88:503–11.
10. Ilahi OA, Swarna U, Hamill RJ, et al. Concomitant crystal and septic arthritis. Orthopedics 1996;19:613–7.
11. Yu KH, Luo SF, Liou LB, et al. Concomitant septic and gouty arthritis: an analysis of 30 cases. Rheumatology (Oxford) 2003;42:1062–6.
12. Galloway JB, Hyrich KL, Mercer LK, et al. Risk of septic arthritis in patients with rheumatoid arthritis and the effect of anti-TNF therapy: results from the British Society for Rheumatology biologics register. Ann Rheum Dis 2011;70:1810–4.
13. Weston VC, Jones AC, Bradbury N, et al. Clinical features and outcome of septic arthritis in a single UK Health District 1982–1991. Ann Rheum Dis 1999;58:214–9.
14. Ross JJ. Septic arthritis. Infect Dis Clin North Am 2005;19:799–817.
15. Goldenberg DL, Cohen AS. Acute infectious arthritis. Am J Med 1976;60:369–77.
16. Edwards SA, Cranfield T, Clarke HJ. Atypical presentation of septic arthritis in the immunosuppressed patient. Orthopedics 2002;25:1089–90.
17. Jones A, Doherty M. ABC of rheumatology: osteoarthritis. BMJ 1995;310:457–60.
18. Dubost JJ, Fis I, Denis P, et al. Polyarticular septic arthritis. Medicine (Baltimore) 1993;72:296–310.
19. Brancos MA, Peris P, Miro JM, et al. Septic arthritis in heroin addicts. Semin Arthritis Rheum 1991;21:81–7.

20. Vyskocil JJ, McIlroy MA, Brennan TA, et al. Pyogenic infection of the sacroiliac joint: case reports and review of the literature. Medicine (Baltimore) 1991;70: 188–97.
21. Zimmermann B III, Mikolich DJ, Lally EV. Septic sacroiliitis. Semin Arthritis Rheum 1996;26:592–604.
22. Ross JJ, Hu LT. Septic arthritis of the pubic symphysis: review of 100 cases. Medicine (Baltimore) 2003;82:340–5.
23. Ross JJ, Shamsuddin H. Sternoclavicular septic arthritis: review of 180 cases. Medicine (Baltimore) 2004;83:139–48.
24. Sharp JT, Lidsky MD, Duffy J, et al. Infectious arthritis. Arch Intern Med 1979;139: 1125–30.
25. Ross JJ, Davidson L. Methicillin-resistant *Staphylococcus aureus* septic arthritis: an emerging clinical syndrome. Rheumatology (Oxford) 2005;44:1197–8.
26. Daynes J, Roth MF, Zekaj M, et al. Adult native septic arthritis in an inner city hospital: effects on length of stay. Orthopedics 2016;39:e674–9.
27. Frazee BW, Fee C, Lambert L. How common is MRSA in adult septic arthritis? Ann Emerg Med 2009;54:695–700.
28. Helito CP, Noffs GG, Pecora JR, et al. Epidemiology of septic arthritis of the knee at Hospital das Clínicas, Universidade de São Paulo. Braz J Infect Dis 2014;18: 28–33.
29. Chao CM, Lai CC, Hsueh PR. Bacteriology of septic arthritis at a regional hospital in southern Taiwan. J Microbiol Immunol Infect 2013;46:241–2.
30. Dubost JJ, Couderc M, Tatar Z, et al. Three-decade trend in the distribution of organisms causing septic arthritis in native joints. Joint Bone Spine 2014;81(5): 438–40.
31. Clerc O, Prod'hom G, Greub G, et al. Adult native septic arthritis: a review of 10 years of experience and lessons for empirical antibiotic therapy. J Antimicrob Chemother 2011;66:1168–73.
32. Farley MM. Group B streptococcal disease in nonpregnant adults. Clin Infect Dis 2001;33:556–61.
33. Dubost JJ, Soubrier M, De Champs C, et al. No changes in the distribution of organisms responsible for septic arthritis over a 20 year period. Ann Rheum Dis 2002;61:267–9.
34. Nolla JM, Gomez-Vaquero C, Corbella X, et al. Group B streptococcus (*Streptococcus agalactiae*) pyogenic arthritis in nonpregnant adults. Medicine (Baltimore) 2003;82:119–27.
35. Li SF, Henderson J, Dickman E, et al. Laboratory tests in adults with monoarticular arthritis: can they rule out a septic joint? Acad Emerg Med 2004;11:276–80.
36. Belkhir L, Rodriguez-Villalobos H, Vandercam B, et al. Pneumococcal septic arthritis in adults: clinical analysis and review. Acta Clin Belg 2014;69:40–6.
37. Pulido M, Sorvillo F. Declining invasive pneumococcal disease mortality in the United States, 1990-2005. Vaccine 2010;28:889–92.
38. O'Brien JP, Goldenberg DL, Rice PA. Disseminated gonococcal infection: a prospective analysis of 49 patients and a review of pathophysiology and immune mechanisms. Medicine (Baltimore) 1983;62:395–406.
39. Goldenberg DL, Brandt KD, Cathcart ES, et al. Acute arthritis due to gram-negative bacilli: a clinical characterization. Medicine (Baltimore) 1974;53: 197–208.
40. Bayer AS, Chow AW, Louie JS, et al. Gram-negative bacillary septic arthritis: clinical, radiographic, therapeutic, and prognostic features. Semin Arthritis Rheum 1977;7:123–32.

41. Newman ED, Davis DE, Harrington TM. Septic arthritis due to gram negative bacilli: older patients with good outcome. J Rheumatol 1988;15:659–62.
42. Schaad UB. Arthritis in disease due to *Neisseria meningitidis*. Rev Infect Dis 1980;2:880–8.
43. Goedvolk CA, von Rosenstiel IA, Bos AP. Immune complex associated complications in the subacute phase of meningococcal disease: incidence and literature review. Arch Dis Child 2003;88:927–30.
44. Rompalo AM, Hook EW III, Roberts PL, et al. The acute arthritis-dermatitis syndrome: the changing importance of *Neisseria gonorrhoeae* and *Neisseria meningitidis*. Arch Intern Med 1987;147:281–3.
45. Armstrong RW, Bolding F, Joseph R. Septic arthritis following arthroscopy: clinical syndromes and analysis of risk factors. Arthroscopy 1992;8:213–23.
46. Indelli PF, Dillingham M, Fanton G, et al. Septic arthritis in postoperative anterior cruciate ligament reconstruction. Clin Orthop 2002;398:182–8.
47. Gardam M, Lim S. Mycobacterial osteomyelitis and arthritis. Infect Dis Clin North Am 2005;19:819–30.
48. Eder L, Zisman D, Rozenbaum M, et al. Clinical features and aetiology of septic arthritis in northern Israel. Rheumatology (Oxford) 2005;44:1559–63.
49. Gotuzzo E, Alarcon GS, Bocanegra TS, et al. Articular involvement in human brucellosis: a retrospective analysis of 304 cases. Semin Arthritis Rheum 1982; 12:245–55.
50. Solera J, Rodriguez-Zapata M, Geijo P, et al. Doxycycline-rifampin versus doxycycline-streptomycin in treatment of human brucellosis due to *Brucella melitensis*. Antimicrob Agents Chemother 1995;39:2061–7.
51. Kratz A, Greenberg D, Barki Y, et al. *Pantoea agglomerans* as a cause of septic arthritis after palm tree thorn injury; case report and literature review. Arch Dis Child 2003;88:542–4.
52. Freiberg AA, Herzenberg JE, Sangeorzan JA. Thorn synovitis of the knee joint with *Nocardia pyarthrosis*. Clin Orthop 1993;287:233–6.
53. Talan DA, Abrahamian FM, Moran GJ, et al. Clinical presentation and bacteriologic analysis of infected human bites in patients presenting to emergency departments. Clin Infect Dis 2003;37:1481–9.
54. Talan DA, Citron DM, Abrahamian FM, et al. Bacteriologic analysis of infected dog and cat bites. N Engl J Med 1999;340:85–92.
55. Chevalier X, Martigny J, Avouac B, et al. Report of 4 cases of *Pasteurella multocida* septic arthritis. J Rheumatol 1991;18:1890–2.
56. Feurle GE, Marth T. An evaluation of antimicrobial treatment for Whipple's disease: tetracycline versus trimethoprim-sulfamethoxazole. Dig Dis Sci 1994;39: 1642–8.
57. Mahnel R, Kalt A, Ring S, et al. Immunosuppressive therapy in Whipple's disease patients is associated with the appearance of gastrointestinal manifestations. Am J Gastroenterol 2005;100:1167–73.
58. Lange U, Teichmann J. Whipple arthritis: diagnosis by molecular analysis of synovial fluid–current status of diagnosis and therapy. Rheumatology (Oxford) 2003;42:473–80.
59. Mahnel R, Marth T. Progress, problems, and perspectives in diagnosis and treatment of Whipple's disease. Clin Exp Med 2004;4:39–43.
60. Asmar BI, Andresen J, Brown WJ. Ureaplasma urealyticum arthritis and bacteremia in agammaglobulinemia. Pediatr Infect Dis J 1998;17:73–6.

61. O'Sullivan MV, Isbel NM, Johnson DW, et al. Disseminated pyogenic *Mycoplasma pneumoniae* infection in a renal transplant recipient, detected by broad-range polymerase chain reaction. Clin Infect Dis 2004;39:e98–9.

62. Mian AN, Farney AC, Mendley SR. Mycoplasma hominis septic arthritis in a pediatric renal transplant recipient: case report and review of the literature. Am J Transplant 2005;5:183–8.

63. Baum C, Hsu JP, Nelson RC. The impact of the addition of naloxone on the use and abuse of pentazocine. Public Health Rep 1987;102:426–9.

64. Darke S, Kaye S, Ross J. Geographic injecting locations among injecting drug users in Sydney, Australia. Addiction 2001;96:241–6.

65. Krogstad P, Smith AL. Osteomyelitis and septic arthritis. In: Feigin RD, Cherry JD, editors. Textbook of pediatric infectious disease. 4th edition. Philadelphia: WB Saunders; 1998. p. 683–704.

66. Luhmann JD, Luhmann SJ. Etiology of septic arthritis in children: an update for the 1990s. Pediatr Emerg Care 1999;15:40–2.

67. Yagupsky P, Peled N, Katz O. Epidemiological features of invasive *Kingella kingae* infections and respiratory carriage of the organism. J Clin Microbiol 2002;40:4180–4.

68. Centers for Disease Control and Prevention. Osteomyelitis/septic arthritis caused by *Kingella kingae* among day care attendees in Minnesota, 2003. MMWR Morb Mortal Wkly Rep 2004;53:241–3.

69. Centers for Disease Control and Prevention. *Kingella kingae* infections in children. United States, June 2001-November 2002. MMWR Morb Mortal Wkly Rep 2004;53:244.

70. Erickson CM, Sue PK, Stewart K, et al. Sequential parenteral to oral clindamycin dosing in pediatric musculoskeletal infection. Pediatr Infect Dis J 2016;35:1092–6.

71. Wang CL, Wang SM, Yang YJ, et al. Septic arthritis in children: relationship of causative pathogens, complications, and outcome. J Microbiol Immunol Infect 2003;36:41–6.

72. Margaretten ME, Kohlwes J, Moore D, et al. Does this adult patient have septic arthritis? JAMA 2007;297:1478–88.

73. Fye KH. Arthrocentesis, synovial fluid analysis, and synovial biopsy. In: Klippel JH, editor. Primer on the rheumatic diseases. 12th edition. Atlanta: Arthritis Foundation; 2001. p. 138–44.

74. McCutchan HJ, Fisher RC. Synovial leukocytosis in infectious arthritis. Clin Orthop 1990;257:226–30.

75. Shmerling RH, Delbanco TL, Tosteson AN, et al. Synovial fluid tests. What should be ordered? JAMA 1990;264:1009–14.

76. Carpenter CR, Schuur JD, Everett WW, et al. Evidence-based diagnostics: adult septic arthritis. Acad Emerg Med 2011;18:781–96.

77. Shen CJ, Wu MS, Lin KH, et al. The use of procalcitonin in the diagnosis of bone and joint infections: a systematic review and meta-analysis. Eur J Clin Microbiol Infect Dis 2013;32:807–14.

78. Paosong S, Narongroeknawin P, Pakchotanon R, et al. Serum procalcitonin as a diagnostic aid in patients with acute bacterial septic arthritis. Int J Rheum Dis 2015;18:353–9.

79. Yagupsky P, Press J. Use of the isolator 1.5 microbial tube for culture of synovial fluid from patients with septic arthritis. J Clin Microbiol 1997;35:2410–2.

80. Hughes JG, Vetter EA, Patel R, et al. Culture with BACTEC Peds Plus/F bottle compared with conventional methods for detection of bacteria in synovial fluid. J Clin Microbiol 2001;39:4468–71.
81. Hepburn MJ, Fraser SL, Rennie TA, et al. Septic arthritis caused by *Granulicatella adiacens*: diagnosis by inoculation of synovial fluid into blood culture bottles. Rheumatol Int 2003;23:255–7.
82. Pääkkönen M, Peltola H. Treatment of acute septic arthritis. Pediatr Infect Dis J 2013 Jun;32(6):684–5.
83. Gupta MN, Sturrock RD, Field M. Prospective comparative study of patients with culture proven and high suspicion of adult onset septic arthritis. Ann Rheum Dis 2003;62:327–31.
84. Pioro MH, Mandell BF. Septic arthritis. Rheum Dis Clin North Am 1997;23:239–58.
85. Smith JW, Piercy EA. Infectious arthritis. Clin Infect Dis 1995;20:225–31.
86. Song HK, Guy TS, Kaiser LR, et al. Current presentation and optimal surgical management of sternoclavicular joint infection. Ann Thorac Surg 2002;73:427–31.
87. Kachala SS, D'Souza DM, Teixeira-Johnson L, et al. Surgical management of sternoclavicular joint infections. Ann Thorac Surg 2016;101:2155–60.
88. Broy SB, Schmid FR. A comparison of medical drainage (needle aspiration) and surgical drainage (arthrotomy or arthroscopy) in the initial treatment of infected joints. Clin Rheum Dis 1986;12:501–22.
89. Odio CM, Ramirez T, Arias G, et al. Double blind, randomized, placebo-controlled study of dexamethasone therapy for hematogenous septic arthritis in children. Pediatr Infect Dis J 2003;22:883–9.
90. Salter RB. The biologic concept of continuous passive motion of synovial joints: the first 18 years of research and its clinical application. Clin Orthop 1989;242: 12–25.

Diagnosis of Prosthetic Joint Infection
Cultures, Biomarker and Criteria

Eric O. Gomez-Urena, MD*, Aaron J. Tande, MD,
Douglas R. Osmon, MD, Elie F. Berbari, MD

KEYWORDS

- Prosthetic joint infection • Arthroplasty • Diagnosis

KEY POINTS

- In patients undergoing revision arthroplasty, infections should always be considered and excluded prior to or at the time of surgery.
- No single diagnostic test has enough accuracy for the detection of prosthetic joint infection; therefore, a combination of preoperative and intraoperative tests is needed for the diagnosis of arthroplasty infection.
- Serologic inflammatory markers are useful tests in selecting patients who would benefit from more invasive procedures such as arthrocentesis.
- The optimization of traditional tissue culture and biofilm-dislodging techniques has improved the identification of the causative agent.
- Synovial fluid measurement of cytokines are promising new emerging tests.

INTRODUCTION

Total joint arthroplasty is a highly successful treatment modality that improves joint function, relieves pain, and increases the overall quality of life.[1] Prosthetic joint infection (PJI) is one of the most dreaded complications of arthroplasties that has been reported in 0.5% to 0.8% of patients undergoing primary total knee and hip arthroplasties.[2] With a projected increase in the number of primary arthroplasties, even at a steady infection rate, more infectious complications are expected in the next decades. The cost of treatment of a PJI is 3 to 4 times the cost of a primary implantation,[3] which imposes a great burden to the health care system. Despite the abilities of curing and/or controlling PJI with current treatment regimens, patients with PJI

Disclosures: The authors have nothing to disclose.
Division of Infectious Diseases, Mayo Clinic School of Medicine, 200 First Street Southwest, Rochester, MN 55905, USA
* Corresponding author. Division of Infectious Diseases, Mayo Clinic, 200 First Street Southwest, Rochester, MN 55905.
E-mail address: Urena.eric@mayo.edu

Infect Dis Clin N Am 31 (2017) 219–235
http://dx.doi.org/10.1016/j.idc.2017.01.008
0891-5520/17/© 2017 Elsevier Inc. All rights reserved.

have inferior functional results compared with patients who undergo revisions for aseptic joint failure.[4]

Even though infection is the most common cause of knee arthroplasty revision and the third most common cause of hip arthroplasty revision[5] in the United States, discriminating between aseptic joint failure and chronic PJI can still be a challenging task. An accurate diagnosis is important, as the therapeutic approach differs between PJI and aseptic failure. Failing to identify a PJI will lead to placement of prosthesis in an infected joint space, which could compromise the outcome of the arthroplasty. On the other hand, misdiagnosis of PJI can lead to unnecessary antimicrobial use and surgical procedures with an increased morbidity and cost to the health care system.

PJIs are biofilm-related infections in which bacteria attach to the inert surface of the prosthesis forming communities embedded within an extracellular polymeric matrix.[6] This biofilm leads to a persistent infection that is maintained by a relative antimicrobial resistance and tolerance to the host defenses (immune reaction). Currently, the presence of PJI is evaluated by detecting the invading organisms (ie, cultures) or by assessing the host immune response to the infection (ie, serologic tests and inflammatory cell counts). Biofilm-related infections are difficult to diagnose, as traditional microbiological tests are optimized to detect free-floating bacteria (planktonic) but not bacteria within the biofilm (sessile). In addition, arthroplasty infections caused by low virulence organisms may fail to illicit a systemic inflammatory response detectable by clinical symptoms or serologic tests.

Several tests with different levels of complexity have been evaluated for the detection of PJI, and none of them have shown an adequate diagnostic accuracy to be used as a stand-alone test. The accuracy of any given test can only be measured by comparing the results of the test to a clearly established definition of disease (gold standard). Such a gold-standard definition of PJI does not currently exist. Different definitions have been used among studies evaluating diagnostic tests for detection of PJI that could compromise the validity and comparability of results. In an effort to standardize the definition of PJI, multiple medical societies and working groups have proposed different definitions. In 2011, the Musculoskeletal Infectious Society (MSIS) proposed a set of criteria for the diagnosis of PJI that was later revised by the International Consensus Meeting on PJI (**Table 1**).[7,8] In 2012, the Infectious Diseases Society of America (IDSA) published a set of criteria for the definition of PJI.[9] These definitions have only minor differences in determining the presence of infection.[6]

CLINICAL PRESENTATION

Clinical presentation of PJI is dependent on the time of onset from prosthesis placement, mechanism of infection, virulence of the pathogen, and host immune response (**Table 2**). History and physical examination can improve the accuracy of diagnostic tests. By carefully selecting patients who would obtain the most benefit from a diagnostic test, one can minimize the false-positive and false-negative results. Numerous tests are currently available to aid physicians in the evaluation of PJI. However, the selection of these tests and the interpretation of their results should be made in conjunction with the likelihood of infection based on history and physical examination.

Joint pain is the most common presentation of PJI and aseptic failure. Joint erythema and systemic signs such as chills and fever are highly specific for infection but are rarely seen except in acute hematogenous PJI or early postoperative infections.[10–14] Other conditions, such as gout, may have a similar presentation with local signs of inflammation in the affected prosthesis. A sinus tract communicating with the

Table 1
Proposed definitions of prosthetic joint infections

IDSA	Musculoskeletal Infection Society (MSIS) 2011	International Consensus Meeting 2013
PJI is present when one of the following criteria is present: • Sinus tract communicating with prosthesis • Presence of purulence • Acute inflammation on histopathologic evaluation of periprosthetic tissue • Two or more positive cultures with same organism (intraoperatively and/or preoperatively) • Single positive culture with virulent organism	PJI is present when one major criteria is present or four out of six minor criteria exist Major Criteria: • Two positive periprosthetic cultures with phenotypically identical organisms • A sinus tract communicating with the joint Minor criteria: • Elevated CRP and ESR • Elevated synovial fluid WBC count or ++ change on leukocyte esterase test strip • Elevated synovial fluid PMN% • Presence of purulence in the affected joint • Positive histologic analysis of periprosthetic tissue • A single positive culture	PJI is present when one major criteria is present or three out of five minor criteria exist Major Criteria: • Two positive periprosthetic cultures with phenotypically identical organisms • A sinus tract communicating with the joint Minor criteria: • Elevated CRP and ESR • Elevated synovial fluid WBC count or ++ change on leukocyte esterase test strip • Elevated synovial fluid PMN% • Positive histologic analysis of periprosthetic tissue • A single positive culture

Abbreviations: CRP, C-reactive protein; ESR, erythrocyte sedimentation rate; PMN%, polymorphonuclear neutrophils percentage.
Adapted from Refs.[7–9]

Table 2
Classification and clinical presentation of prosthetic joint infections

Type of Infection	Time to Presentation	Mechanism of Infection	Organisms	Clinical Presentation	
Early	<3 mo	Intraoperative contamination	Virulent bacteria (ie, *Staphylococcus aureus*)	Acute	Sudden onset erythema, edema, warmth, and tenderness
Delayed	3–12 mo	Intraoperative contamination	Low virulent bacteria (coagulase-negative staphylococci)	Chronic	Joint pain and stiffness
Late	>12 mo	Hematogenous seeding	Virulent bacteria (ie, *S.aureus*)	Acute	Sudden-onset erythema, edema, warmth, and tenderness
		Intraoperative contamination	Low virulent bacteria (ie, *Propionibacterium acnes*)	Chronic	Joint pain, sinus tract

Adapted from Parvizi J, Fassihi SC, Enayatollahi MA. Diagnosis of periprosthetic joint infection following hip and knee arthroplasty. Orthop Clin North Am 2016;47(3):509; with permission.

prosthesis is one of the most specific signs of PJI and by itself has been considered diagnostic.[10] It is important to assess for postoperative wound healing complications such as prolonged wound drainage, wound dehiscence, wound hematoma, or lack of resolution of joint pain after primary surgery.[15] Imaging studies showing early implant loosening (<5 years from implantation) may also be a presentation of PJI. Risk factors associated with PJI include prolonged operative time, immunosuppression, previous arthroplasty, and history of prior surgical site infection. Presence of these risk factors may raise the index of suspicion for PJI.

The Mayo Prosthetic Joint Risk Score has been proposed as a prognostic scoring system that could also be applied in the diagnostic process of PJI. This scoring system encompasses preoperative (body mass index, prior surgeries, prior arthroplasty, immunosuppression, American Society of Anesthesiologists (ASA) score), intraoperative (procedure time), and postoperative (wound dehiscence, infection, hematoma, deep organ infection) variables to identify high-risk patients with higher pretesting probability of PJI.[16] Once a clinical suspicion for PJI has been established (pretest probability of infection), clinicians can use further diagnostic tests to increase or decrease the likelihood of a PJI in a patient (**Fig. 1**).

PREOPERATIVE EVALUATION

Prior to a revision arthroplasty, an earnest attempt to detect PJI should be made in order to formulate an optimal therapeutic strategy. Several preoperative tests are available to assist physicians in the assessment of PJI.

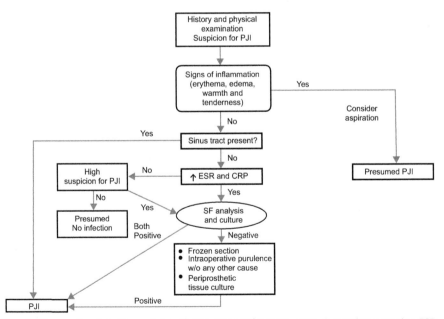

Fig. 1. Diagnostic algorithm of prosthetic joint infections. CRP, C-reactive protein; ESR, erythrocyte sedimentation rate; PJI, prosthetic joint infection; SF, synovial fluid; w/o, without. (*Adapted from* Osmon DR, Berbari EF, Berendt AR, et al. Diagnosis and management of prosthetic joint infection: clinical practice guidelines by the Infectious Diseases Society of America. Clin Infect Dis 2013;56(1):e3; with permission.)

White Blood Cell Count and Serologic Tests

White blood cell (WBC) count lacks sensitivity (45%) to detect PJI and is rarely helpful in the evaluation of PJI[17]; therefore it is not recommended.

Erythrocyte sedimentation rate (ESR) and C-reactive protein (CRP) are inexpensive, widely available, noninvasive and low complexity tests that have now been incorporated in the routine evaluation of PJI. An arbitrary threshold of greater than 30 mm/h for ESR and greater than 10 mg/L for C-reactive protein (CRP) have been proposed for the diagnosis of PJI.[7,18] In a meta-analysis, ESR and CRP showed a pooled sensitivity of 75% and 88% and a pooled specificity of 70% and 74%, respectively.[17] The combined use of ESR and CRP had a sensitivity of 96%, indicating that if both tests are negative, infection is unlikely.[19,20] In a large retrospective study at the Mayo Clinic, a normal ESR ($\leq$30 mm/h) and CRP ($\leq$10 mg/L) were able to predict the absence of infection in 94% of patients with total knee arthroplasty and total hip arthroplasty (THA) infections.[21] However, PJI may be rarely present in patients with normal levels of ESR and CRP. A recent retrospective study reported that 4% of PJI (by MSIS criteria) had negative ESR and CRP.[19,20] Infections with low virulent organisms, prior antimicrobial use, and immunosuppression have been suggested as possible factors associated with normal inflammatory markers.[19]

The major drawback of ESR/CRP is the limited specificity. Elevation of ESR has been associated with concomitant noninfectious causes such as renal disease, malignancy, chronic inflammatory conditions, and advanced age, among others.[22] Although CRP is more specific than ESR, it may also be elevated in inflammatory conditions, infections, and neoplasia.[17]

Synovial Fluid Cell Count and Culture

Diagnostic arthrocentesis should be performed whenever there is suspicion of PJI to assess synovial fluid cell counts, polymorphonuclear leukocyte percentage (PMN%), and synovial fluid culture. The selection of patients who would benefit from arthrocentesis should be based on history and physical examination along with inflammatory marker results (elevated ESR and CRP).[23]

Because of the superficial location of the knee joint compared with the hip, orthopedic surgeons are more prone to aspirate the knee joint in the office setting. Hip arthrocentesis is usually performed through an imaging-guided technique by interventional radiology. If a dry tap is encountered where no fluid is aspirated, normal saline can be injected into the joint and reaspirated for synovial fluid culture only. With the injection of normal saline, cell counts may not be accurate.[24] The specificity of cultures obtained through saline injection may be lower.[24] The amount of synovial fluid obtained during aspiration does not correlate with the presence or absence of infection.

Different cutoffs for synovial fluid WBC counts have been recommended for diagnosis of PJI, but these are much lower than those reported for native septic arthritis. Cell counts and PMN% thresholds are different for TKA infection (1100–3000 cell/μL and 64%–75%)[20,25–27] than THA infection (745–3000 cells/μL and 73.5%–80%).[28,29] The MSIS PJI definition proposed a standard synovial fluid cell count of greater than 3000 cells/μL and PMN% greater than 80% as suggestive of hip or knee arthroplasty infection. These cutoff values for synovial fluid cell count and PMN% apply only to prostheses that have been implanted more than 3 to 6 months. If this criterion is applied to arthroplasties placed during the first 90 days, it could lead to false-positive results (>25%).[30] Therefore, in the early postoperative period (within the first 6 weeks after implantation) a higher synovial fluid cell count cutoff of at least 10,700 cells/μL and 89% PMN%, or a total neutrophil count of greater than

10,000 cells/μL has been proposed for detection of acute PJI.[30,31] Despite the different cutoff proposed for synovial WBC and PMN%, a recent meta-analysis showed a pooled sensitivity and specificity for the detection of PJI of 88% and 93% for synovial WBC and 90% and 88% for PMN%, respectively.[32]

Synovial cell counts may be elevated in periprosthetic fractures, inflammatory arthritis, and allergy to metal. However, a recent study suggested that synovial fluid cell count and PMN% might perform similarly in patients with inflammatory arthritis as in patients without inflammatory arthritis.[11] Although total cell count may be spuriously elevated in metal-on-metal failure when using an automated cell counter, the neutrophil percentage appears to have preserved accuracy to discriminate infection from this condition.[33]

Synovial fluid should also be sent for microbial culture, as its results could assist in the preoperative selection of antimicrobials added to the cement spacer and in the immediate postoperative period. Discordance between synovial fluid cultures and intraoperative cultures has been reported, with false-positive results between 5% and 13%.[12,15,34] The use of automated blood culture systems has improved the sensitivity and specificity of the synovial fluid culture when compared with agar plate cultures. Automated blood culture systems seem to result in greater identification of pathogens and fewer contaminants in native joint septic arthritis and in PJI.[35] The better specificity could be due to less risk of contamination during processing compared with agar plates.

By combining results of synovial fluid cell count, differential diagnosis, and culture to ESR and CRP, the sensitivity to detect PJI can be improved up to 99.7%.[19] In a systematic review of the several studies, synovial fluid cultures had a pooled sensitivity, specificity, positive likelihood ratio, and negative likelihood ratio of 0.72 (0.65–0.78), 0.95 (0.93–0.97), 15.3 (10.6–22.1), and 0.29 (0.23–0.38), respectively, to predict presence of PJI.[36]

INTRAOPERATIVE EVALUATION

In selected patients, PJI cannot be confirmed or excluded in the preoperative period, and infection will not be detected until after the arthroplasty revision is performed. Visual inspection of joint and histopathological examination of periprosthetic tissue samples through frozen sections can assist surgeons in the intraoperative assessment of infection while the patient is still in the operating room. Periprosthetic tissue culture results, although valuable, are only available after the surgical revision.

Periprosthetic Purulence

Conventionally, presence of periprosthetic purulence has been considered as definitive evidence of PJI. However, with concerns of the subjective interpretation of purulence (frank pus vs turbid synovial fluid) other noninfectious causes of aseptic failure that can induce a purulent-like fluid response, recent studies have questioned the reliability of intraoperative purulence as a single criterion for diagnosis of PJI.[8,37] Intraarticular purulence can occur in crystal-induced arthritis, reaction to metal debris from metal-on-metal prosthesis, or metal corrosion in THA. In the absence of other causes of purulence, the IDSA guidelines consider intraoperative purulence a diagnostic criterion for PJI.[9]

Histopathology

Periprosthetic tissue can be sent for histopathological determination of acute inflammation. Different thresholds for acute inflammation have been proposed, but presence of at least 5 to 10 PMN per high-power field (×400 magnification) in at least 5 microscopic fields is one of the most common definitions used. Histopathology evaluation has a high specificity in predicting culture positive PJI and therefore confirming the presence of infection.[38] However, a major drawback of frozen section is the limited sensitivity reported in some studies (18%–67%).[39–44] Sampling bias, pathologist expertise, and infections caused by low virulent organisms (ie, *Proprionibacterium acnes*) that fail to induce a neutrophilic reaction[38,45,46] may contribute to the low sensitivity reported in some studies. Intraoperative frozen sections can provide useful information to surgeons at the time of the revision surgery, bearing in mind that inflammatory arthritis and periprosthetic fracture may also give false-positive results.[47]

Periprosthetic Tissue Cultures

Multiple periprosthetic tissue samples should be collected and submitted for cultures. Antimicrobial agents should be held until cultures are collected if the patient is not systemically ill. The number of cultures needed for optimal detection of pathogens is unknown, but several studies recommend at least 4 to 6 samples (periprosthetic tissue and synovial fluid).[48,49] As common pathogens of PJI are also part of the normal skin flora, multiple tissue samples are needed not only to improve the sensitivity but also to optimize the specificity by aiding in the distinction of a contaminant from a pathogen. Isolation of the same organism (based on phenotype) from multiple cultures suggests the presence of PJI.[50] Nevertheless, a single positive culture for a virulent organism (ie, *Staphylococcus aureus* or gram-negative organism) should be carefully evaluated and not discarded immediately as a contaminant.[51]

Although Gram stain from periprosthetic tissue has a high specificity (>97%), the low sensitivity (0%–27%) makes it rarely helpful in ruling out PJI; therefore, it is not routinely recommended.[6] Swab cultures have a lower sensitivity and specificity compared with tissue cultures, and they are not recommended.[52,53] Inoculation of periprosthetic tissues into blood culture bottles seems to provide a higher sensitivity and faster results when compared with cultures using conventional plates and broth media.[49,54,55] The incubation time of periprosthetic cultures is debatable, but some authors advocate for extended incubation of cultures to improve sensitivity.[55] Extended incubation (at least 14 days) is especially important for anaerobic cultures, as it significantly improves recovery of *P acnes*.[55,56] One concern about prolonging incubation time is the potential of enhancing the recovery of contaminants. However, Schäfer and colleagues[57] reported that half of the contaminating strains were detected within 7 days of incubation. These findings suggest that there is no increased risk to detect contaminant with prolonged incubation, but further studies are needed to determine optimal incubation time of periprosthetic cultures.

PJI caused by mycobacteria and fungi is rare; therefore, routine use mycobacterial and fungal periprosthetic tissue cultures is not cost-effective.[58] The mycobacterial and fungal cultures should be performed based on the clinical suspicion for these infections, epidemiology data, and host immune status (ie, immunosuppressed patients). The MSIS and IDSA do not recommend routine mycobacterial and fungal cultures.

Sonicate Cultures

In an effort to improve the sensitivity of periprosthetic tissue cultures for the microbiological diagnosis of PJI, dislodgement of the biofilm from the prosthesis using vortex/sonication has been proposed. Trampuz and colleagues[59] reported that sonicate fluid cultures detected more pathogens (78.5%) compared with periprosthetic tissue cultures (60.8%), especially in patients with prior antimicrobial use (75% in sonicate fluid vs 45% in tissue culture). Sonicate fluid cultures also detect microbial growth earlier than tissue cultures.[60] A resent meta-analysis showed a pooled sensitivity and specificity of 80% and 95%, respectively.[61] However, despite the higher sensitivity of sonicate fluid cultures, sonication of the prosthesis has not been widely adopted in routine clinical practice because of the complexity and added cost of the test.

Culture-Negative Prosthetic Joint Infections

Absence of bacterial growth has been reported in up to 14% of patients with clinical evidence of PJI.[6] Significant numbers of culture-negative PJI appear to be caused by prior antimicrobial exposure.[62,63] Inability to identify an etiologic pathogen in PJI can also be caused by infections due to mycobacteria, fungi, and fastidious bacteria (ie, zoonosis) that are not detected by routine bacterial cultures and require specialized culture media or serologic assays for the detection of antibodies or antigens.[64] In a literature review, Million and colleagues[65] reported that of 301 cases of culture-negative PJI, 46% were due to fungi, 43% to mycobacteria, and 11% to bacteria. Inadequate numbers of samples and a slow growth pattern caused by phenotypic changes of bacteria within the biofilm may also influence the recovery of pathogens. Lastly, it is important to recognize that other noninfectious conditions may mimic arthroplasty infection, and they could be misdiagnosed as culture-negative PJI. Conditions such as gout, metal-on-metal arthroplasty failure, or trunnion corrosion, when appropriate, should be considered in the differential diagnosis of culture-negative PJI.[66]

When faced with a culture-negative PJI, physicians should consider the following approach to optimize the microbiological diagnosis. In patients being evaluated for PJI who are receiving or have recently received antimicrobial therapy, microbiological evaluation should be delayed until after antimicrobial agents are discontinued (if clinically feasible). The optimal duration of the antimicrobial washout period is unknown, but a minimum of 2 weeks is recommended to improve the bacterial recovery rate. If synovial fluid cultures obtained by aspiration are negative, a repeat aspiration of the joint should be attempted. Multiple periprosthetic tissue samples should be collected and extended incubation of cultures should be considered to identify slow growing organisms (*P acnes*). If the periprosthetic aerobic and anaerobic bacterial cultures are negative, fungal and mycobacterial cultures should be requested and added to the initial cultures. Sonication of the explanted prosthesis should be considered as it has been shown to detect more pathogens when compared with tissue cultures, especially when patients have been exposed to antimicrobials prior to collection of cultures.[59] Additional microbiological diagnostic evaluation (ie, serology or special culture media) should be performed based on epidemiologic risk factors such as travel history or environmental or animal exposure to rule out unusual organisms such as *Coxiella burnetti* or *Brucella species*.[67,68] Molecular tests may be useful and can be considered if available.

ADVANCEMENTS IN PROSTHETIC JOINT INFECTION DIAGNOSTICS: NOVEL TESTS
Molecular Tests

Culture-negative PJIs pose a great challenge in terms of management, so new laboratory methods that improve the microbiological diagnosis of PJI are well desired. Infections caused by fastidious organisms, lack of viability during transport, or prior antimicrobial use could be factors associated with culture-negative infections. Molecular methods could overcome these limitations with the added advantage of improved turn-around-time that could potentially be useful as a point-of-care test during intraoperative assessment.[69] Broad-range 16S rRNA polymerase chain reaction (PCR),[70] genus-/group-specific PCR,[71] PCR-electrospray ionization mass spectrometry[72] on synovial fluid,[73] and periprosthetic tissue[74] or sonicate fluid cultures have been evaluated. Molecular tests using sonicate fluid have shown improved sensitivity compared with routine periprosthetic tissue and sonicate fluid cultures[72] but not when applied to tissue samples.[74,75] Molecular tests also have inherent limitations such as risk for false-positive results from DNA contamination, lack of antimicrobial susceptibility results, and inability to identify all organisms present in polymicrobial infections.[70,71] These limitations, along with the added cost and test complexity, have hindered the wide adoption of molecular tests in clinical practice.

Synovial Fluid Leukocyte Esterase Strip Test

Leukocyte esterase (LE) is an enzyme present within neutrophils that is locally secreted at the site of an infection. LE strip test is a colorimetric strip test that measures (semiquantitative) the presence and amount of LE. This test is routinely used in the assessment of urinary tract infection, but Parvizi and colleagues[76] reported its use on synovial fluid for the detection of TKA PJI. The test has a reported sensitivity of 79.2% to 100% and specificity of 80.8% to 93%, with great correlation to synovial PMN results.[76–80] This test has an added advantage over synovial fluid cell count as it provides faster results (1–2 minutes) that could potentially allow its use intraoperatively as a point-of-care test. Also, it is associated with low cost and possible higher sensitivity than synovial WBC, as it measures LE from dead and ruptured WBCs that would have been missed by cell count. Its major utility is in ruling out infection with a negative LE test (negative/trace) based on consistent high negative predictive values reported. Blood and metal debris associated with implant failure may give unreadable and false-positive results, but recent studies showed that LE is highly specific even in metal debris-associated implant failure.[66] Bloody synovial fluid invalidates the use of the LE strip, as it interferes with the color reading of the test strip, but centrifugation of the synovial fluid seems to allow the use of LE test in these cases.[79] This test may not be useful in the postoperative assessment of PJI, as it may be overly sensitive, leading to false-positive results, but this has not been studied in this setting.

Serum Interleukin-6

Interleukin-6 (IL-6) is a cytokine produced by monocytes and macrophages that has been shown to be useful in the diagnosis of PJI. Ettinger and colleagues[81] demonstrated that IL-6 (cutoff of 5.12 pg/mL) had a diagnostic odds ratio of 28.6 compared with 7.1 for CRP, but in a combined diagnostic algorithm using IL-6 and CRP, the diagnostic odds ratio improved to 168. In a meta-analysis, IL-6 was shown to have a higher diagnostic odds ratio (314.69) when compared with ESR and CRP.[17]

Synovial Fluid Biomarkers

In the last few years, there has been a growing interest in synovial fluid biomarkers for the diagnosis of PJI. Since PJIs are infections mainly confined to the joint, one would expect that the host inflammatory response would be more enhanced at the local site than systemically; therefore, measurement of biomarkers in synovial fluid could be theoretically more sensitive in detecting PJI than when measured in serum. Likewise, synovial fluid biomarkers would not be impacted by other nonjoint-related inflammatory conditions or infections improving the specificity. Different cytokines, inflammatory proteins, and antimicrobial peptides have been evaluated as potential synovial fluid biomarkers that could correctly identify patients with PJI in a timely manner.

Alpha-defensin (α-defensin 1–3)

Alpha-defensins are small antimicrobial peptides primarily detected within the azurophilic granules of neutrophils (also called human neutrophil peptides). Defensins, as part of the innate immune system, have antimicrobial activity against a wide variety of organisms.[82] Deirmengian and colleagues[83] evaluated a panel of synovial fluid biomarkers in 95 patients with THA and TKA for the diagnosis of PJI by MSIS criteria. Chronic inflammatory conditions and antimicrobial use at the time of aspiration were not criteria for exclusion. In this study, alpha-defensin, BPI, ELA-2, lactoferrin, and NGAL were shown to be 100% sensitive and specific for the diagnosis of PJI. The same authors optimized the alpha-defensin immunoassay to detect extracellular alpha-defensin 1-3 on synovial fluid.[84] Several studies have shown that synovial fluid alpha-defensin has a high sensitivity (97%–100%) and high specificity (95%–100%) for detection of PJI.[84–88]

As the alpha-defensin test does not seem to correlate with the synovial WBC count, it could be useful in patients with inflammatory arthritis or other chronic inflammatory conditions.[83,85] However, metallosis might result in a false-positive alpha-defensin test.[88] The results from these studies are encouraging and are indicative that alpha-defensin may improve the detection of PJI in clinical practice. The utility of alpha-defensin in patients with low virulent infections (P acnes, coagulase-negative Staphylococcus) and in patients with nonhip or nonknee joint infections, as well as the cost effectiveness as compared with standard diagnostic approaches, have not been fully evaluated.

Synovial interleukin-6

Synovial fluid IL-6 level has been shown to be more specific than serum IL-6 level in the diagnosis of PJI. Randau and colleagues[89] showed that synovial IL-6 level (cutoff >2100 pg/mL) had sensitivity and specificity of 62.5% and 85.7%, respectively for the diagnosis of PJI. Lenski and Scherer[90] reported the use of synovial IL-6 in diagnosis of PJI (knees, hips, and elbows) with a sensitivity and specificity of 90% and 94.7%, respectively, using a cutoff of at least 30,750 pg/mL. Further studies are required to validate these finding before synovial IL-6 can be brought to clinical practice.

Synovial C-reactive protein

Serum levels of CRP seem to correlate with synovial fluid levels of CRP.[91] Synovial fluid CRP seems to perform better and add to the diagnosis of PJI when compared with serum CRP.[92–94] A recent meta-analysis showed that synovial fluid CRP had a diagnostic odds ratio of 101.4,[95] which was much higher than the value of 13.1 reported for serum CRP in a different meta-analysis.[17] This meta-analysis included studies that used different testing platforms for the detection of synovial CRP as well as different cutoff. Further studies should be performed, especially to determine specific cutoff to be used in clinical practice.

Shoulder and Elbow Arthroplasty Infections

Diagnosing PJI after shoulder arthroplasty infection can be an arduous task. The current diagnostic armamentarium for PJI has been extensively studied, optimized, and used for the diagnosis of hip and knee arthroplasty infections, but may not be as accurate in shoulder and elbow arthroplasties. The most common pathogens isolated from infected shoulder arthroplasties are low virulence organisms such P acnes and coagulase-negative staphylococci. It appears that these organisms induce a lesser host immune response that results in clinically indolent infection difficult to diagnose.

Shoulder arthroplasty infection

The most common presentation of patients with shoulder arthroplasty infections is joint pain and stiffness.[96,97] Local and systemic symptoms and signs of infection are rare. ESR and CRP are less sensitive in shoulders than in knees and hips, with sensitivities of 16% and 42% reported in 1 study, respectively.[21] This low sensitivity limits its utility as a screening test for detection of PJI. Arthrocentesis has been recommended in the evaluation of a painful shoulder arthroplasty. However, the accuracy, utility, and threshold for synovial fluid cell count have not been fully evaluated in prosthetic shoulders. Preoperative synovial fluid cultures have been reported to be positive between 50% to 93% of patients with PJI of the shoulder.[96–100] Diagnostic arthroscopy with periprosthetic tissue biopsy and cultures appears to be more sensitive than synovial fluid aspiration and culture. In a recent study, arthroscopic tissue biopsy identified pathogens more often than synovial fluid culture collected through arthrocentesis.[101]

Histopathologic examination of periprosthetic tissue, employing the same criteria for acute inflammation used in knees and hips, has a low sensitivity (50%–63%) but similar specificity.[96,102] However, a different cutoff (a total of 10 PMN in 5 high-power-field) seems to improve the sensitivity (70%) without affecting specificity.[101]

Serum IL-6 is a poor predictor for positive tissue cultures at time of revision shoulder arthroplasty with sensitivity of 12% to 14% but with higher positive predictive value (67%) compared with ESR and CRP.[103,104] In contrast, a recent study indicates that measurement of synovial IL-6 may be more helpful than serum IL-6, with a reported sensitivity and specificity of 87% and 90%, respectively.[105] Along the same lines, synovial fluid alpha-defensin was reported to predict shoulder PJI with a sensitivity and specificity of 63% and 95%, respectively.[106] The performance of these tests in shoulder PJI appears to be inferior when compared with hip or knee PJI.

Elbow arthroplasty infection

Less is known about the performance of established diagnostic tests in patients with suspected elbow PJI. The elbow is a superficially located joint with a minimal amount of soft tissue around it. Thus, signs of inflammation are more apparent when compared with hips and knees. Scattered reports suggest that ESR and CRP perform similarly, and histopathology has a lower sensitivity for detection of elbow PJI compared with hips or knees PJI.[107–109] To the authors' knowledge, there are no studies evaluating the use of arthrocentesis or any of the emerging new tests for the diagnosis of PJI in the elbow.

SUMMARY

Major contributions in the advancements of PJI diagnostics have been made in recent years. Nevertheless, all of the current diagnostic tests have inherent limitations that will still require the combination of different testing modalities to assist clinicians in the diagnosis of PJI. New assays are needed not only for the detection of PJI but also for pathogen identification so that appropriate antimicrobial therapy can be provided. While waiting for the advent of new technologies, clinical judgment, above all tests, should guide the physician's decision making to accurately differentiate aseptic arthroplasty failure and PJI.

REFERENCES

1. Jones CA, Voaklander DC, Johnston DW, et al. Health related quality of life outcomes after total hip and knee arthroplasties in a community based population. J Rheumatol 2000;27(7):1745–52.

2. Phillips JE, Crane TP, Noy M, et al. The incidence of deep prosthetic infections in a specialist orthopaedic hospital: a 15-year prospective survey. J Bone Joint Surg Br 2006;88(7):943–8.

3. Hebert CK, Williams RE, Levy RS, et al. Cost of treating an infected total knee replacement. Clin Orthop Relat Res 1996;(331):140–5.

4. Barrack RL, Engh G, Rorabeck C, et al. Patient satisfaction and outcome after septic versus aseptic revision total knee arthroplasty. J Arthroplasty 2000; 15(8):990–3.

5. Bozic KJ, Kamath AF, Ong K, et al. Comparative epidemiology of revision arthroplasty: failed THA poses greater clinical and economic burdens than failed TKA. Clin Orthop Relat Res 2015;473(6):2131–8.

6. Tande AJ, Patel R. Prosthetic joint infection. Clin Microbiol Rev 2014;27(2): 302–45.

7. Parvizi J, Zmistowski B, Berbari EF, et al. New definition for periprosthetic joint infection: from the Workgroup of the Musculoskeletal Infection Society. Clin Orthop Relat Res 2011;469(11):2992–4.

8. Parvizi J, Gehrke T. International Consensus Group on Periprosthetic Joint I. Definition of periprosthetic joint infection. J Arthroplasty 2014;29(7):1331.

9. Osmon DR, Berbari EF, Berendt AR, et al. Diagnosis and management of prosthetic joint infection: clinical practice guidelines by the Infectious Diseases Society of America. Clin Infect Dis 2013;56(1):e1–25.

10. Tsaras G, Osmon DR, Mabry T, et al. Incidence, secular trends, and outcomes of prosthetic joint infection: a population-based study, Olmsted County, Minnesota, 1969-2007. Infect Control Hosp Epidemiol 2012;33(12):1207–12.

11. Cipriano CA, Brown NM, Michael AM, et al. Serum and synovial fluid analysis for diagnosing chronic periprosthetic infection in patients with inflammatory arthritis. J Bone Joint Surg Am 2012;94(7):594–600.

12. Lachiewicz PF, Rogers GD, Thomason HC. Aspiration of the hip joint before revision total hip arthroplasty. Clinical and laboratory factors influencing attainment of a positive culture. J Bone Joint Surg Am 1996;78(5):749–54.

13. Duff GP, Lachiewicz PF, Kelley SS. Aspiration of the knee joint before revision arthroplasty. Clin Orthop Relat Res 1996;(331):132–9.

14. Teller RE, Christie MJ, Martin W, et al. Sequential indium-labeled leukocyte and bone scans to diagnose prosthetic joint infection. Clin Orthop Relat Res 2000;(373):241–7.

15. Barrack RL, Harris WH. The value of aspiration of the hip joint before revision total hip arthroplasty. J Bone Joint Surg Am 1993;75(1):66–76.

16. Berbari EF, Osmon DR, Lahr B, et al. The Mayo prosthetic joint infection risk score: implication for surgical site infection reporting and risk stratification. Infect Control Hosp Epidemiol 2012;33(8):774–81.

17. Berbari E, Mabry T, Tsaras G, et al. Inflammatory blood laboratory levels as markers of prosthetic joint infection: a systematic review and meta-analysis. J Bone Joint Surg Am 2010;92(11):2102–9.

18. Alijanipour P, Bakhshi H, Parvizi J. Diagnosis of periprosthetic joint infection: the threshold for serological markers. Clin Orthop Relat Res 2013;471(10):3186–95.

19. McArthur BA, Abdel MP, Taunton MJ, et al. Seronegative infections in hip and knee arthroplasty: periprosthetic infections with normal erythrocyte sedimentation rate and C-reactive protein level. Bone Joint J 2015;97-B(7):939–44.

20. Parvizi J, Ghanem E, Sharkey P, et al. Diagnosis of infected total knee: findings of a multicenter database. Clin Orthop Relat Res 2008;466(11):2628–33.

21. Piper KE, Fernandez-Sampedro M, Steckelberg KE, et al. C-reactive protein, erythrocyte sedimentation rate and orthopedic implant infection. PLoS One 2010;5(2):e9358.
22. Levine SE, Esterhai JL Jr, Heppenstall RB, et al. Diagnoses and staging. Osteomyelitis and prosthetic joint infections. Clin Orthop Relat Res 1993;(295): 77–86.
23. Gould ES, Potter HG, Bober SE. Role of routine percutaneous hip aspirations prior to prosthesis revision. Skeletal Radiol 1990;19(6):427–30.
24. Ali F, Wilkinson JM, Cooper JR, et al. Accuracy of joint aspiration for the preoperative diagnosis of infection in total hip arthroplasty. J Arthroplasty 2006;21(2): 221–6.
25. Ghanem E, Parvizi J, Burnett RS, et al. Cell count and differential of aspirated fluid in the diagnosis of infection at the site of total knee arthroplasty. J Bone Joint Surg Am 2008;90(8):1637–43.
26. Trampuz A, Hanssen AD, Osmon DR, et al. Synovial fluid leukocyte count and differential for the diagnosis of prosthetic knee infection. Am J Med 2004; 117(8):556–62.
27. Zmistowski B, Restrepo C, Huang R, et al. Periprosthetic joint infection diagnosis: a complete understanding of white blood cell count and differential. J Arthroplasty 2012;27(9):1589–93.
28. Chalmers PN, Sporer SM, Levine BR. Correlation of aspiration results with periprosthetic sepsis in revision total hip arthroplasty. J Arthroplasty 2014;29(2): 438–42.
29. Schinsky MF, Della Valle CJ, Sporer SM, et al. Perioperative testing for joint infection in patients undergoing revision total hip arthroplasty. J Bone Joint Surg Am 2008;90(9):1869–75.
30. Christensen CP, Bedair H, Della Valle CJ, et al. The natural progression of synovial fluid white blood-cell counts and the percentage of polymorphonuclear cells after primary total knee arthroplasty: a multicenter study. J Bone Joint Surg Am 2013;95(23):2081–7.
31. Bedair H, Ting N, Jacovides C, et al. The Mark Coventry Award: diagnosis of early postoperative TKA infection using synovial fluid analysis. Clin Orthop Relat Res 2011;469(1):34–40.
32. Qu X, Zhai Z, Liu X, et al. Evaluation of white cell count and differential in synovial fluid for diagnosing infections after total hip or knee arthroplasty. PLoS One 2014;9(1):e84751.
33. Wyles CC, Larson DR, Houdek MT, et al. Utility of synovial fluid aspirations in failed metal-on-metal total hip arthroplasty. J Arthroplasty 2013;28(5):818–23.
34. Fehring TK, Cohen B. Aspiration as a guide to sepsis in revision total hip arthroplasty. J Arthroplasty 1996;11(5):543–7.
35. Hughes JG, Vetter EA, Patel R, et al. Culture with BACTEC Peds Plus/F bottle compared with conventional methods for detection of bacteria in synovial fluid. J Clin Microbiol 2001;39(12):4468–71.
36. Qu X, Zhai Z, Wu C, et al. Preoperative aspiration culture for preoperative diagnosis of infection in total hip or knee arthroplasty. J Clin Microbiol 2013;51(11): 3830–4.
37. Alijanipour P, Adeli B, Hansen EN, et al. Intraoperative purulence is not reliable for diagnosing periprosthetic joint infection. J Arthroplasty 2015;30(8):1403–6.
38. Tsaras G, Maduka-Ezeh A, Inwards CY, et al. Utility of intraoperative frozen section histopathology in the diagnosis of periprosthetic joint infection: a systematic review and meta-analysis. J Bone Joint Surg Am 2012;94(18):1700–11.

39. Fehring TK, McAlister JA Jr. Frozen histologic section as a guide to sepsis in revision joint arthroplasty. Clin Orthop Relat Res 1994;(304):229–37.

40. Abdul-Karim FW, McGinnis MG, Kraay M, et al. Frozen section biopsy assessment for the presence of polymorphonuclear leukocytes in patients undergoing revision of arthroplasties. Mod Pathol 1998;11(5):427–31.

41. Della Valle CJ, Bogner E, Desai P, et al. Analysis of frozen sections of intraoperative specimens obtained at the time of reoperation after hip or knee resection arthroplasty for the treatment of infection. J Bone Joint Surg Am 1999;81(5):684–9.

42. Musso AD, Mohanty K, Spencer-Jones R. Role of frozen section histology in diagnosis of infection during revision arthroplasty. Postgrad Med J 2003;79(936):590–3.

43. Frances Borrego A, Martinez FM, Cebrian Parra JL, et al. Diagnosis of infection in hip and knee revision surgery: intraoperative frozen section analysis. Int Orthop 2007;31(1):33–7.

44. Ko PS, Ip D, Chow KP, et al. The role of intraoperative frozen section in decision making in revision hip and knee arthroplasties in a local community hospital. J Arthroplasty 2005;20(2):189–95.

45. Bori G, Munoz-Mahamud E, Garcia S, et al. Interface membrane is the best sample for histological study to diagnose prosthetic joint infection. Mod Pathol 2011;24(4):579–84.

46. Grosso MJ, Frangiamore SJ, Ricchetti ET, et al. Sensitivity of frozen section histology for identifying *Propionibacterium acnes* infections in revision shoulder arthroplasty. J Bone Joint Surg Am 2014;96(6):442–7.

47. Shah RP, Plummer DR, Moric M, et al. Diagnosing infection in the setting of periprosthetic fractures. J Arthroplasty 2016;31(9 Suppl):140–3.

48. Atkins BL, Athanasou N, Deeks JJ, et al. Prospective evaluation of criteria for microbiological diagnosis of prosthetic-joint infection at revision arthroplasty. The OSIRIS Collaborative Study Group. J Clin Microbiol 1998;36(10):2932–9.

49. Bemer P, Leger J, Tande D, et al. How many samples and how many culture media to diagnose a prosthetic joint infection: a clinical and microbiological prospective multicenter study. J Clin Microbiol 2016;54(2):385–91.

50. DeHaan A, Huff T, Schabel K, et al. Multiple cultures and extended incubation for hip and knee arthroplasty revision: impact on clinical care. J Arthroplasty 2013;28(8 Suppl):59–65.

51. Saleh A, Guirguis A, Klika AK, et al. Unexpected positive intraoperative cultures in aseptic revision arthroplasty. J Arthroplasty 2014;29(11):2181–6.

52. Font-Vizcarra L, Garcia S, Martinez-Pastor JC, et al. Blood culture flasks for culturing synovial fluid in prosthetic joint infections. Clin Orthop Relat Res 2010;468(8):2238–43.

53. Aggarwal VK, Higuera C, Deirmengian G, et al. Swab cultures are not as effective as tissue cultures for diagnosis of periprosthetic joint infection. Clin Orthop Relat Res 2013;471(10):3196–203.

54. Minassian AM, Newnham R, Kalimeris E, et al. Use of an automated blood culture system (BD BACTEC) for diagnosis of prosthetic joint infections: easy and fast. BMC Infect Dis 2014;14:233.

55. Peel TN, Dylla BL, Hughes JG, et al. Improved diagnosis of prosthetic joint infection by culturing periprosthetic tissue specimens in blood culture bottles. MBio 2016;7(1). e01776–15.

56. Butler-Wu SM, Burns EM, Pottinger PS, et al. Optimization of periprosthetic culture for diagnosis of propionibacterium acnes prosthetic joint infection. J Clin Microbiol 2011;49(7):2490–5.

57. Schafer P, Fink B, Sandow D, et al. Prolonged bacterial culture to identify late periprosthetic joint infection: a promising strategy. Clin Infect Dis 2008;47(11): 1403–9.

58. Wadey VM, Huddleston JI, Goodman SB, et al. Use and cost-effectiveness of intraoperative acid-fast bacilli and fungal cultures in assessing infection of joint arthroplasties. J Arthroplasty 2010;25(8):1231–4.

59. Trampuz A, Piper KE, Jacobson MJ, et al. Sonication of removed hip and knee prostheses for diagnosis of infection. N Engl J Med 2007;357(7):654–63.

60. Dailey A, Nyre L, Piper KE, et al. Hip or knee prosthesis sonicate cultures have a shorter time to positivity compared to periprosthetic tissue cultures. In: Abstracts of the Interscience Conference on Antimicrobial Agents and Chemotherapy (ICAAC) 49th Annual Meeting American Society for Microbiology, San Francisco, CA, September 12-15, 2009.

61. Zhai Z, Li H, Qin A, et al. Meta-analysis of sonication fluid samples from prosthetic components for diagnosis of infection after total joint arthroplasty. J Clin Microbiol 2014;52(5):1730–6.

62. Malekzadeh D, Osmon DR, Lahr BD, et al. Prior use of antimicrobial therapy is a risk factor for culture-negative prosthetic joint infection. Clin Orthop Relat Res 2010;468(8):2039–45.

63. Berbari EF, Marculescu C, Sia I, et al. Culture-negative prosthetic joint infection. Clin Infect Dis 2007;45(9):1113–9.

64. Marculescu CE, Berbari EF, Cockerill FR 3rd, et al. Fungi, mycobacteria, zoonotic and other organisms in prosthetic joint infection. Clin Orthop Relat Res 2006;451:64–72.

65. Million M, Bellevegue L, Labussiere AS, et al. Culture-negative prosthetic joint arthritis related to Coxiella burnetii. Am J Med 2014;127(8):786.e7-10.

66. Tischler EH, Plummer DR, Chen AF, et al. Leukocyte esterase: metal-on-metal failure and periprosthetic joint infection. J Arthroplasty 2016;31(10):2260–3.

67. Tande AJ, Cunningham SA, Raoult D, et al. A case of Q fever prosthetic joint infection and description of an assay for detection of Coxiella burnetii. J Clin Microbiol 2013;51(1):66–9.

68. Weil Y, Mattan Y, Liebergall M, et al. Brucella prosthetic joint infection: a report of 3 cases and a review of the literature. Clin Infect Dis 2003;36(7):e81–86.

69. Vasoo S, Cunningham SA, Greenwood-Quaintance KE, et al. Evaluation of the FilmArray blood culture ID panel on biofilms dislodged from explanted arthroplasties for prosthetic joint infection diagnosis. J Clin Microbiol 2015;53(8): 2790–2.

70. Gomez E, Cazanave C, Cunningham SA, et al. Prosthetic joint infection diagnosis using broad-range PCR of biofilms dislodged from knee and hip arthroplasty surfaces using sonication. J Clin Microbiol 2012;50(11):3501–8.

71. Cazanave C, Greenwood-Quaintance KE, Hanssen AD, et al. Rapid molecular microbiologic diagnosis of prosthetic joint infection. J Clin Microbiol 2013; 51(7):2280–7.

72. Greenwood-Quaintance KE, Uhl JR, Hanssen AD, et al. Diagnosis of prosthetic joint infection by use of PCR-electrospray ionization mass spectrometry. J Clin Microbiol 2014;52(2):642–9.

73. Melendez DP, Greenwood-Quaintance KE, Berbari EF, et al. Evaluation of a Genus- and Group-Specific Rapid PCR assay panel on synovial fluid for diagnosis of prosthetic knee infection. J Clin Microbiol 2016;54(1):120–6.

74. Ryu SY, Greenwood-Quaintance KE, Hanssen AD, et al. Low sensitivity of periprosthetic tissue PCR for prosthetic knee infection diagnosis. Diagn Microbiol Infect Dis 2014;79(4):448–53.

75. Bemer P, Plouzeau C, Tande D, et al. Evaluation of 16S rRNA gene PCR sensitivity and specificity for diagnosis of prosthetic joint infection: a prospective multicenter cross-sectional study. J Clin Microbiol 2014;52(10):3583–9.

76. Parvizi J, Jacovides C, Antoci V, et al. Diagnosis of periprosthetic joint infection: the utility of a simple yet unappreciated enzyme. J Bone Joint Surg Am 2011; 93(24):2242–8.

77. Shafafy R, McClatchie W, Chettiar K, et al. Use of leucocyte esterase reagent strips in the diagnosis or exclusion of prosthetic joint infection. Bone Joint J 2015;97-B(9):1232–6.

78. Wetters NG, Berend KR, Lombardi AV, et al. Leukocyte esterase reagent strips for the rapid diagnosis of periprosthetic joint infection. J Arthroplasty 2012;27(8 Suppl):8–11.

79. Aggarwal VK, Tischler E, Ghanem E, et al. Leukocyte esterase from synovial fluid aspirate: a technical note. J Arthroplasty 2013;28(1):193–5.

80. Tischler EH, Cavanaugh PK, Parvizi J. Leukocyte esterase strip test: matched for musculoskeletal infection society criteria. J Bone Joint Surg Am 2014; 96(22):1917–20.

81. Ettinger M, Calliess T, Kielstein JT, et al. Circulating biomarkers for discrimination between aseptic joint failure, low-grade infection, and high-grade septic failure. Clin Infect Dis 2015;61(3):332–41.

82. Suarez-Carmona M, Hubert P, Delvenne P, et al. Defensins: "simple" antimicrobial peptides or broad-spectrum molecules? Cytokine Growth Factor Rev 2015; 26(3):361–70.

83. Deirmengian C, Kardos K, Kilmartin P, et al. Diagnosing periprosthetic joint infection: has the era of the biomarker arrived? Clin Orthop Relat Res 2014; 472(11):3254–62.

84. Deirmengian C, Kardos K, Kilmartin P, et al. The alpha-defensin test for periprosthetic joint infection outperforms the leukocyte esterase test strip. Clin Orthop Relat Res 2015;473(1):198–203.

85. Deirmengian C, Kardos K, Kilmartin P, et al. Combined measurement of synovial fluid alpha-defensin and C-reactive protein levels: highly accurate for diagnosing periprosthetic joint infection. J Bone Joint Surg Am 2014;96(17): 1439–45.

86. Bingham J, Clarke H, Spangehl M, et al. The alpha defensin-1 biomarker assay can be used to evaluate the potentially infected total joint arthroplasty. Clin Orthop Relat Res 2014;472(12):4006–9.

87. Frangiamore SJ, Gajewski ND, Saleh A, et al. α-defensin accuracy to diagnose periprosthetic joint infection-best available test? J Arthroplasty 2016;31(2): 456–60.

88. Bonanzinga T, Zahar A, Dutsch M, et al. How reliable is the alpha-defensin immunoassay test for diagnosing periprosthetic joint infection? A prospective study. Clin Orthop Relat Res 2016;475(2):408–15.

89. Randau TM, Friedrich MJ, Wimmer MD, et al. Interleukin-6 in serum and in synovial fluid enhances the differentiation between periprosthetic joint infection and aseptic loosening. PLoS One 2014;9(2):e89045.

90. Lenski M, Scherer MA. The significance of interleukin-6 and lactate in the synovial fluid for diagnosing native septic arthritis. Acta Orthop Belg 2014;80(1): 18–25.

91. Parvizi J, McKenzie JC, Cashman JP. Diagnosis of periprosthetic joint infection using synovial C-reactive protein. J Arthroplasty 2012;27(8 Suppl):12–6.

92. Ronde-Oustau C, Diesinger Y, Jenny JY, et al. Diagnostic accuracy of intra-articular C-reactive protein assay in periprosthetic knee joint infection–a preliminary study. Orthop Traumatol Surg Res 2014;100(2):217–20.

93. Omar M, Ettinger M, Reichling M, et al. Synovial C-reactive protein as a marker for chronic periprosthetic infection in total hip arthroplasty. Bone Joint J 2015; 97-B(2):173–6.

94. Parvizi J, Jacovides C, Adeli B, et al. Coventry award: synovial C-reactive protein: a prospective evaluation of a molecular marker for periprosthetic knee joint infection. Clin Orthop Relat Res 2012;470(1):54–60.

95. Wang C, Wang Q, Li R, et al. Synovial fluid C-reactive protein as a diagnostic marker for periprosthetic joint infection: a systematic review and meta-analysis. Chin Med J (Engl). 2016;129(16):1987–93.

96. Sperling JW, Kozak TK, Hanssen AD, et al. Infection after shoulder arthroplasty. Clin Orthop Relat Res 2001;(382):206–16.

97. Coste JS, Reig S, Trojani C, et al. The management of infection in arthroplasty of the shoulder. J Bone Joint Surg Br 2004;86(1):65–9.

98. Strickland JP, Sperling JW, Cofield RH. The results of two-stage re-implantation for infected shoulder replacement. J Bone Joint Surg Br 2008;90(4):460–5.

99. Sabesan VJ, Ho JC, Kovacevic D, et al. Two-stage reimplantation for treating prosthetic shoulder infections. Clin Orthop Relat Res 2011;469(9):2538–43.

100. Ince A, Seemann K, Frommelt L, et al. One-stage exchange shoulder arthroplasty for peri-prosthetic infection. J Bone Joint Surg Br 2005;87(6):814–8.

101. Dilisio MF, Miller LR, Warner JJ, et al. Arthroscopic tissue culture for the evaluation of periprosthetic shoulder infection. J Bone Joint Surg Am 2014;96(23): 1952–8.

102. Jawa A, Shi L, O'Brien T, et al. Prosthesis of antibiotic-loaded acrylic cement (PROSTALAC) use for the treatment of infection after shoulder arthroplasty. J Bone Joint Surg Am 2011;93(21):2001–9.

103. Villacis D, Merriman JA, Yalamanchili R, et al. Serum interleukin-6 as a marker of periprosthetic shoulder infection. J Bone Joint Surg Am 2014;96(1):41–5.

104. Grosso MJ, Frangiamore SJ, Saleh A, et al. Poor utility of serum interleukin-6 levels to predict indolent periprosthetic shoulder infections. J Shoulder Elbow Surg 2014;23(9):1277–81.

105. Frangiamore SJ, Saleh A, Kovac MF, et al. Synovial fluid interleukin-6 as a predictor of periprosthetic shoulder infection. J Bone Joint Surg Am 2015;97(1): 63–70.

106. Frangiamore SJ, Saleh A, Grosso MJ, et al. α-defensin as a predictor of periprosthetic shoulder infection. J Shoulder Elbow Surg 2015;24(7):1021–7.

107. Gille J, Ince A, Gonzalez O, et al. Single-stage revision of peri-prosthetic infection following total elbow replacement. J Bone Joint Surg Br 2006;88(10): 1341–6.

108. Morrey BF, Bryan RS. Infection after total elbow arthroplasty. J Bone Joint Surg Am 1983;65(3):330–8.

109. Ahmadi S, Lawrence TM, Morrey BF, et al. The value of intraoperative histology in predicting infection in patients undergoing revision elbow arthroplasty. J Bone Joint Surg Am 2013;95(21):1976–9.

Management of Prosthetic Joint Infection

Aaron J. Tande, MD*, Eric O. Gomez-Urena, MD, Elie F. Berbari, MD,
Douglas R. Osmon, MD

KEYWORDS

- Prosthetic joint infection • Periprosthetic joint infection • Osteomyelitis
- Joint arthroplasty • 2-Stage exchange • Joint replacement • Septic arthritis

KEY POINTS

- Although definitive cure of prosthetic joint infection (PJI) may not always be possible, alleviation of the symptoms of PJI and restoration of function should always be the goal.
- Successful treatment involves débridement of infected tissue, explicit management of the prosthesis, and pathogen-directed antimicrobial treatment tailored to the specific surgical approach.
- The choice of medical/surgical strategy depends on chronicity of infection, condition of the joint and implant, and patient ability and desire to undergo 1 or more surgeries.

INTRODUCTION

Joint arthroplasty has improved life for millions of people around the world. The benefits of this procedure include restoration of function and relief of pain. Fortunately, the incidence of peri-PJI or PJI is low. When it does occur, PJI is a challenging condition to treat. The purpose of this review is to provide an overview of the management of PJI.

GENERAL PRINCIPLES AND TREATMENT SUCCESS

In its simplest form, the goal of medicine is to cure disease afflicting a patient. For a PJI, this ideally means eradication of infection and resolution of the symptoms associated with infection, ultimately leading to freedom from further therapy.[1] In reality, "cure" may not be an achievable goal for all patients. Therefore, the goals of PJI treatment (and the corresponding definition of treatment success) should take into account patient preferences and may align more closely with the concept of disease control rather than cure, thus seeking to minimize the impact of PJI on the quality and quantity

Disclosure Statement: The authors have nothing to disclose.
Division of Infectious Diseases, Department of Internal Medicine, Mayo Clinic, 200 1st Street Southwest, Rochester, MN 55905, USA
* Corresponding author.
E-mail address: tande.aaron@mayo.edu

Infect Dis Clin N Am 31 (2017) 237–252
http://dx.doi.org/10.1016/j.idc.2017.01.009
0891-5520/17/© 2017 Elsevier Inc. All rights reserved.

id.theclinics.com

of a patient's life. For example, the most common single symptom of PJI is pain.[2] Accordingly, relief of pain must be of paramount importance but is not the only consideration. Other priorities, such as restoration of function, avoidance of further surgical interventions, and freedom from antimicrobial suppression, may be of varying degrees of importance to individual patients. An open and honest discussion of realistic treatment goals help guide the choice of medical and surgical approach.

There are several different surgical treatment strategies that are described in this review. Each of these strategies has identical components: (1) débride all infected tissue; (2) minimize or eliminate the impact of the prosthesis on perpetuating biofilm-related infection, either by complete resection of the prosthesis or exchange of the removable components; and (3) maintain sufficient soft tissue coverage to permit healing. These are similar to the principles of surgical osteomyelitis management described by Dr J. Albert Key more than 70 years ago.[3] Coordination with a plastic surgeon may be needed to achieve dead space management and soft tissue coverage, particularly in the setting of hip arthroplasty infection and multiply revised joints, respectively. A conceptual overview of the different medical/surgical treatment strategies is shown in **Fig. 1**.[4]

Successful medical therapy begins with an accurate microbiologic diagnosis of the cause of the infection to permit the most effective, safe, and narrow spectrum of antimicrobial therapy. Reported antimicrobial allergies should be investigated thoroughly, and patients with reported penicillin allergy should undergo allergy consultation and penicillin skin testing to make available all necessary antimicrobial therapy. The choice and duration of antimicrobial therapy should be modified according to the surgical approach (discussed later; see **Fig. 1**). Development of and coordination with an outpatient antimicrobial therapy program are critical to monitor for and minimize antimicrobial treatment-related side effects.[5] In addition, there are antimicrobial-related adverse effects that are unique to prolonged antimicrobial use, such as minocycline skin change.[6] Providers managing long-term PJI treatment must be aware of these effects and discuss them with patients. The authors' strategy for monitoring for adverse effects associated with oral antimicrobials is to perform complete blood cell count with differential, liver function testing, and serum creatinine measurement every 2 weeks for 1 month, monthly for 2 months, and yearly thereafter.

SELECTION OF A MEDICAL/SURGICAL STRATEGY

Several factors must be considered when determining an appropriate treatment strategy, including the duration of symptoms, the stability of the implant, the condition of the soft tissue and bone stock, presence of systemic infection symptoms, patient comorbidities, ability or desire to undergo multiple surgeries, patient preferences, and the pathogen causing the infection. The acuity of the symptoms, in conjunction with the availability of surgical expertise, also determines the strategy. If the most appropriate surgical strategy is beyond the capability of the available orthopedic surgeon, then referral to a higher level of care is indicated. Several different algorithms have been published to guide clinicians to appropriate surgical strategy, based on these factors.[7–10] These algorithms may help identify patients who may be likely to have a good outcome with a single surgery, such as débridement, antibiotics, and implant retention (DAIR) or 1-stage exchange (OSE),[11] an approach supported by the literature.[12,13] The algorithm in the IDSA guidelines may also help identify patients in whom a 2-stage exchange (TSE) is less appropriate than alternative approaches, such as permanent resection or arthrodesis, amputation, or medical therapy alone.[9] A modified version of this algorithm is shown in **Fig. 2**.[9]

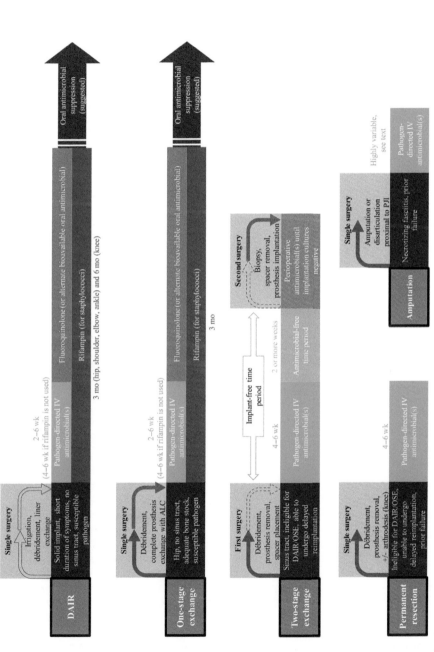

Fig. 1. Medical/surgical treatment strategies. Outlined arrows indicate exchange of polyethylene components only; solid arrows indicate exchange of all arthroplasty components; and dotted arrows indicate exchange of cement spacer. Suppressive oral antimicrobials should immediately follow the 4-week to 6-week course of pathogen-directed therapy, when rifampin-based combination therapy is not used. IV, intravenous. (*Reprinted from* Tande AJ, Patel R. Prosthetic joint infection. Clin Microbiol Rev 2014;27(2):324; with permission.)

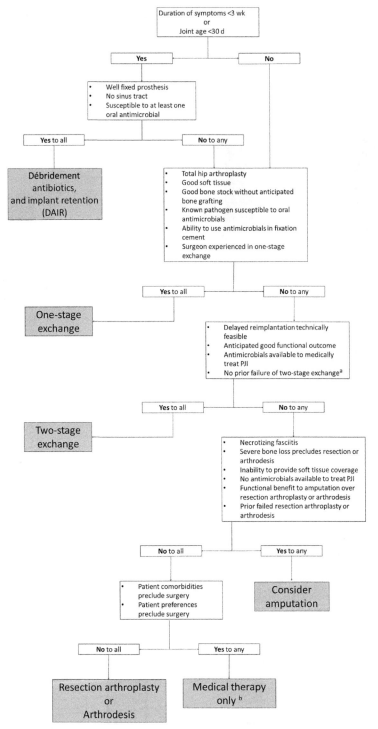

Fig. 2. Algorithm for selection of medical/surgical treatment strategy. Different medical/surgical treatment strategies are shown in the gray boxes. [a] Patients who have previously failed a TSE for other PJIs or for a defined reason could be considered for a second attempt at TSE. [b] Medical therapy only should be reserved for selected cases, as discussed in the text. (*Adapted from* Osmon DR, Berbari EF, Berendt AR, et al. Diagnosis and management of prosthetic joint infection: clinical practice guidelines by the Infectious Diseases Society of America. Clin Infect Dis 2013;56(1):e1–25.)

TWO-STAGE ARTHROPLASTY EXCHANGE

Also known as a staged exchange, TSE involves at least 2 surgeries, typically carried out over several months. In the first surgery (stage 1), after microbiologic and pathologic samples are taken, a thorough débridement is performed and all components and cement are removed, typically followed by placement of a spacer made of high-dose antimicrobial-loaded cement (ALC). After a 4-week to 6-week period of pathogen-directed antimicrobial therapy, patients are monitored off antimicrobials for any signs of ongoing infection, through the use of serial clinical examinations, serum inflammatory markers, and sometimes synovial fluid aspiration. Suspected or demonstrated persistent infection is managed by repeat débridement and further antimicrobials. Once infection is thought to be eradicated, a repeat arthrotomy is performed and the joint is assessed for signs of any infection. If the initial operative inspection and frozen histopathology (if available) are negative for signs of ongoing infection, a new prosthesis is implanted (stage 2), and the cultures that were obtained are monitored under the cover of antimicrobial therapy.

A careful and deliberate approach to the timing of reimplantation (stage 2) is important for a successful outcome, but it is often difficult to tell if infection is eradicated preoperatively or even intraoperatively. A short-interval TSE, when reimplantation is performed within 2 weeks of resection, is associated with a low likelihood of success and generally should be avoided.[14] Some investigators, however, have proposed short-interval TSE as a reasonable strategy.[10] Strategies, such as joint aspiration after antimicrobial holiday[15] and serial measurement of serum[16,17] or synovial fluid inflammatory markers,[18] may provide some information preoperatively but are inaccurate for predicting failure. Acute inflammation on frozen section histopathology at the time of reimplantation is insensitive but highly specific for subsequent failure and persistent infection.[19] Taken collectively, there is no single test that can be done preoperatively or at the time of reimplantation that can definitively rule out persistent infection. All of the available data, however, must be critically assessed at the time of potential reimplantation. The authors' approach is to routinely obtain serum erythrocyte sedimentation rate and C-reactive protein preoperatively and intraoperative frozen section histopathology to guide reimplantation versus débridement with spacer exchange.

TSE is generally considered the most definitive procedure for eradicating infection and restoring function. This strategy is appropriate in the setting of loose prostheses, impaired soft tissue (including sinus tracts), bone loss requiring bone grafting, or infection with organisms, such as mycobacteria, fungi, or drug-resistant bacteria, for which effective suppressive antimicrobial therapy is impossible. The use of high-dose ALC spacers achieves local antimicrobial concentrations much higher than expected using systemic antimicrobial therapy[20,21] and can provide structural stability and better joint space management between the first and second stages of surgery. There are insufficient data, however, to definitively conclude that ALC spacers provide additional benefit in eradication of infection, but, given the structural benefits, the use is generally favored. One recent systematic review found no association between the amount of antimicrobials included in the spacer and control of infection.[22] Contraindications to TSE include the inability and/or unwillingness to undergo multiple surgeries, insufficient bone stock to permit reimplantation with a new arthroplasty, or patients with a baseline functional status where reimplantation would not have a positive impact on outcome, such as patients who are nonambulatory for other reasons.

The antimicrobial treatment strategy that accompanies a TSE procedure is similar to that used for débrided osteomyelitis. Accordingly, most patients receive a 4-week to 6-week course of pathogen-directed intravenous antimicrobials (**Table 1**).[9] When ALC spacers are used, some investigators have reported using oral antimicrobials,[23] a very short duration of antimicrobials,[24] or no systemic antimicrobials.[25] These studies should be cautiously interpreted, however, given that they contained a small number of likely carefully selected patients and that the radical débridement described in one of the studies may not be possible in all institutions.[25] In contrast, there are emerging data that antimicrobial therapy after reimplantation may be beneficial, even if cultures at time of reimplantation are negative. The best data for this approach are from interim analysis of a multicenter randomized trial with 107 patients with hip or knee PJI.[26] The rate of treatment failure was significantly lower among patients randomized to receive 3 months of oral antibiotics compared with those receiving no further antibiotics after reimplantation (5% vs 19%, respectively). These data echo findings from a previous small study using a 28-day course of antibiotics after reimplantation.[27] These data provide some support for giving a limited course of therapy after reimplantation in those patients deemed at high risk for treatment failure or who would have a poor outcome (ie, amputation) with failure. Further studies will hopefully clarify the role of routine oral antimicrobials after reimplantation.

The expected success rate with TSE is generally considered greater than 85% for both hip and knee arthroplasty infection, based on several systematic reviews[28,29] and studies reporting results 5 or more years after treatment.[23,30] Few data suggest that TSE for shoulder PJI has a similar or better outcome with success rate greater than 90%,[31] whereas elbow PJI may have a short-term success rate as low as 72%.[32] Limitations in most of these studies are nonstandardized definition for success and often short follow-up time period.

Risk factors for treatment failure that have been observed in studies of TSE include abnormalities localized to the extremity, such as lymphedema with knee arthroplasty infection,[33] presence of a sinus tract,[12,34] and prior joint revision.[35,36] Comorbid rheumatoid arthritis has also been observed to carry an elevated risk of treatment failure compared with patients without rheumatoid arthritis.[36,37] Finally, although methicillin-resistant *Staphylococcus aureus* (MRSA) has been associated with an increased risk of treatment failure in some studies,[34] an association between the infecting pathogen and likelihood of treatment failure has not been consistently observed.[33,35,38]

It is critically important to recognize that many patients who experience treatment failure after TSE actually suffer reinfection with a new organism, rather than relapse of infection. In one study looking at this question, more than two-thirds of patients who suffered microbiologic failure had infection with a different organism.[39] This finding underscores the importance of approaching each patient encounter as an infection prevention opportunity, at the time of reimplantation arthroplasty. Modifiable risk factors that are associated with infection, such as diabetes mellitus,[40] tobacco abuse,[41] obesity,[42] malnutrition,[43] and screening for and decolonization of S aureus, should all be addressed. Risk scores are available to help quantify the risk of reinfection after revision and may be useful to counsel patients regarding modification of risk factors.[43] Patients should be encouraged to maintain good dental care and minimize any edema, skin breaks, or dermatitis on the limb ipsilateral to the arthroplasty. Antimicrobials may also be loaded into the cement used for arthroplasty reimplantation, with a lower dose typically used to maintain structural stability while providing some benefit of local antimicrobials. In summary, just as the risk of reinfection becomes higher after revision arthroplasty, so too should the intensity of the efforts to prevent infection.

Table 1
Suggested antimicrobials for management of prosthetic joint infection

Microorganism	Preferred Initial Treatment[a]	Alternate Initial Treatment[a]	Initial Combination Therapy	Suppressive Therapy
Staphylococci, methicillin susceptible	Cefazolin or nafcillin	Vancomycin, daptomycin, or oxazolidinone	Rifampin for DAIR and OSE	Cefadroxil, cephalexin, dicloxacillin
Staphylococci, methicillin resistant	Vancomycin	Daptomycin or oxazolidinone	Rifampin for DAIR and OSE	Trimethoprim/sulfamethoxazole, minocycline, doxycycline
Enterococci, penicillin susceptible	Penicillin or ampicillin	Vancomycin, daptomycin, or oxazolidinone	Consider aminoglycoside or ceftriaxone	Penicillin, amoxicillin
Enterococci, penicillin resistant	Vancomycin	Daptomycin or oxazolidinone	Consider aminoglycoside	Linezolid, some may be minocycline susceptible
Pseudomonas aeruginosa	Cefepime or meropenem	Ciprofloxacin or ceftazidime	Consider	Ciprofloxacin
Enterobacter species	Cefepime or ertapenem	Ciprofloxacin	No	Trimethoprim/sulfamethoxazole, ciprofloxacin
Enterobacteriaceae	β-Lactam or ciprofloxacin		No	Trimethoprim/sulfamethoxazole, β-lactam
β-Hemolytic streptococci	Penicillin or ceftriaxone	Vancomycin	No	Penicillin, amoxicillin, cefadroxil
Propionibacterium acnes	Penicillin or ceftriaxone	Vancomycin	No	Penicillin, amoxicillin, cefadroxil

Suggested dosing for normal renal function is from Osmon and colleagues.[9]
[a] Initial antimicrobials are to be given intravenously, except ciprofloxacin or linezolid.
Adapted from Osmon DR, Berbari EF, Berendt AR, et al. Diagnosis and management of prosthetic joint infection: clinical practice guidelines by the Infectious Diseases Society of America. Clin Infect Dis 2013;56(1):e1–25.

ONE-STAGE ARTHROPLASTY EXCHANGE

The OSE procedure involves complete resection of the arthroplasty, a thorough débridement of all infected tissue in the hands of an experienced surgeon, and reimplantation of a new arthroplasty using low-dose ALC, all performed in a single procedure. This strategy is more frequently performed outside the United States. Appropriate patient identification is critical to this strategy.[9] Patients who are eligible for OSE include those with hip PJI, adequate bone stock, an infecting pathogen susceptible to oral antimicrobials and ALC antimicrobials, and an appropriate soft tissue envelope.[8,9] Although small studies have reported success in other situations, such as with bone grafting,[44] knee PJI,[45] and sinus tracts,[46] these remain situations in which TSE is favored.

The antimicrobial approach accompanying OSE is similar to that used with DAIR, using a sequential induction and suppression approach. Although multiple different strategies have been described in the literature, the approach favored by the authors includes 4 weeks to 6 weeks of intravenous or highly bioavailable oral antimicrobial therapy, followed by indefinite chronic oral antimicrobial suppression.[9] There is debate among experts about whether or not long-term suppression is needed, particularly in the setting of staphylococcal infection treated with rifampin-based therapy and gram-negative infection treated with fluoroquinolone therapy.[9]

The success rate for treating PJI with OSE is similar to that of TSE and superior to DAIR. Unfortunately, this statement must be heavily qualified, given that there have been no randomized trials comparing these approaches and there is significant inter-center variability about the preferred approach. A systematic review of hip PJI analyzing 375 patients undergoing OSE reported an 87% success rate, compared with 90% for the 929 patients undergoing TSE.[28] Studies reporting mid-term (5-year) or late (10-year) success rates suggest freedom from infection in greater than 90% of patients with hip PJI.[44,47,48] This approach is used less frequently in knee PJI[45] or shoulder PJI[49] and is not favored by the authors. There have been insufficient studies delineating the risk factors for treatment failure after OSE, but some of the previously discussed risk factors for treatment failure after TSE are postulated to also apply in this situation.

DÉBRIDEMENT WITH IMPLANT RETENTION

Most commonly referred to as a DAIR, this strategy is also known as débridement with prosthesis retention, débridement and component retention, or simply irrigation and débridement. This procedure should be performed with open arthrotomy, such that thorough irrigation and débridement of any necrotic or infected soft tissue can be performed and any hematoma or purulence can be evacuated. Stability of the prosthesis is assessed intraoperatively and any exchangeable components, such as the polyethylene liner or a modular femoral head, should be replaced. The entire joint is then aggressively irrigated and closed.

This strategy is most appropriate in patients with acute infection, either due to hematogenous infection (with symptoms less than 3 weeks) or early postoperative infection (occurring within the first month). Accordingly, patients with a prolonged duration of symptoms, an unstable implant, or a sinus tract, all features expected with a chronic infection, should not be treated with DAIR.[8–10,50] A pathogen that is resistant to all oral antimicrobials is a contraindication to DAIR and should prompt the use of a TSE strategy, but this is often not known at the time of surgery.

As with each of the medical/surgical treatment strategies, antimicrobials are typically withheld preoperatively, except in the setting of systemic infection. Immediately postoperatively, broad-spectrum parenteral antimicrobial therapy is typically indicated, given that the prosthesis is retained and local ALC is not used. After cultures have matured, pathogen-directed therapy is typically given parenterally for the first 2 weeks to 6 weeks.[51–54] The Infectious Diseases Society of America treatment guidelines suggest 4 weeks to 6 weeks of intravenous therapy when rifampin-based combination therapy is not used.[9]

After completion of the initial course of parenteral therapy (or the rifampin combination therapy for staphylococcal infection), many patients are placed on suppressive oral antimicrobial therapy, but this practice is not universal. The use of suppressive therapy has been considered part of the definition of treatment failure in some studies,[55] highlighting the variation in this practice and in the definition of treatment failure in the literature. The optimal duration of suppressive therapy is not clear, with some investigators opting for the first several months after surgery, whereas indefinite suppression is suggested by others. Indefinite suppression for all patients undergoing DAIR results in unnecessary antimicrobial exposure in many patients and the inherent risks therein. The challenge lies in determining in whom antimicrobials can be safely discontinued and when to do so. Although there is no definitive answer to this question, there are some data that may be extrapolated to inform the risk of antimicrobial discontinuation. The largest single study of 345 episodes of *S aureus* PJI treated with DAIR was published in 2013.[55] Important factors when interpreting this Spanish study include a very high rate of rifampin usage (88%) and a very low rate of suppression (5%). Patients with hematogenous infection (as opposed to postsurgical infection), delayed initial débridement, and multiple débridements were all associated with a significantly increased risk of failure after therapy on multivariate analysis. These data suggest that patients with these characteristics should be placed on suppression after completing their course of therapy. Whether the reverse is true, that patients with postsurgical PJI who require only a single promptly performed débridement and are treated with rifampin-based therapy do not need suppression, is not clear. Patients with methicillin-susceptible *S aureus* (MSSA) infection were less likely to fail during therapy but significantly more likely (on univariate analysis) to fail after therapy. It is also not clear whether the findings seen in this study apply to other organisms. An informed discussion with patients about the potential for and consequence of relapse of infection should be part of the decision-making process.

Several characteristics of the microbiology, host, and procedure have been identified as risk factors for treatment failure after DAIR. Infection with *Staphylococcus* species,[52,53,56–58] vancomycin-resistant enterococci,[59] and fluoroquinolone-resistant gram-negative bacilli[60] have all been associated with an overall increased risk of treatment failure compared with other organisms. Systemic patient factors, including cumulative comorbidities, reflected by a high American Society of Anesthesiologists score,[58] or immunocompromised host status[50,55] may also increase the risk for treatment failure. Local host factors specific to the joint or limb, including prior revision[52] and presence of a sinus tract,[50,53] increase the risk of failure, whereas the presence of radiolucency surrounding a mechanically stable implant does not.[53,61] Finally, procedural factors, such as arthroscopic DAIR[52] or a delay until time of surgery,[53,62] are associated with increased risk of failure.

RESECTION WITHOUT REIMPLANTATION AND ARTHRODESIS

Although not a treatment of choice for most patients, resection without reimplantation may be the only therapeutic strategy for some patients. This may be considered when resection is needed for management of infection, but reimplantation with a new arthroplasty via a TSE does not offer a significant functional improvement, such as patients who are limited to a wheelchair for other reasons. This strategy may also be chosen for patients who cannot or do not want a second surgery but require resection for control of the infection or patients in whom a second-stage procedure is forgone due to persistent infection or operative risk. Definitive resection of a hip arthroplasty resulting in a pseudoarthrosis (Girdlestone procedure) is effective at pain relief and infection control but can be expected to lead to significant limb length discrepancies.[63] The use of articulating ALC spacers as destination therapy likely reduces the need for this procedure. Patients who remain with an articulating ALC spacer indefinitely may have a reasonable functional and clinical outcome, based on few available data.[64] Although uncommonly performed after hip arthroplasty resection, knee arthrodesis or fusion may provide additional mechanical stability and the ability to ambulate. Arthrodesis using external fixation may lead to a lower rate of recurrent infection than with an intramedullary nailing,[65] but both methods have advantages and disadvantages. Four weeks to 6 weeks of pathogen-specific antimicrobial therapy is typically used after resection, similar to that for TSE procedures.[9] Demonstration of persistent infection at the time of arthrodesis or suspicion of infected arthrodesis nonunion is typically managed with suppressive oral antimicrobial therapy pending fusion.

AMPUTATION

A vast majority of cases of PJI can be treated successfully with one of the strategies described previously and do not require amputation. Amputation may be considered, however, in the setting of failure of all other therapeutic options[66] or treatment of acute life-threatening infection, such as necrotizing fasciitis,[67] or if it is thought to have a functional benefit for a patient compared with another method of treatment. Unfortunately, a majority of patients who require above-the-knee amputation after knee PJI never become ambulatory again.[66,68] Referral for a second opinion prior to proceeding with amputation is warranted. Appropriate antimicrobial therapy for patients undergoing amputation requires a careful and detailed evaluation of the location of infection, the characteristics of the prosthesis that was amputated, and the procedure performed. Residual osteomyelitis, such as in the acetabulum after a hip disarticulation or in the proximal intramedullary canal of the femur after above the knee amputation, requires treatment of chronic osteomyelitis, whereas amputation with no residual osteomyelitis requires treatment only for possible residual soft tissue infection. As with any treatment of PJI, communication between the infectious diseases physician and the orthopedic surgeon is critical.

ANTIMICROBIAL THERAPY IN SPECIFIC SITUATIONS

The duration, route, and choice of antimicrobial therapy depend the medical/surgical strategy, pathogen(s), comorbidities, and allergies, among other factors. A review of treatments of each of the many possible causes of PJI is beyond scope of this review but has been previously discussed in other comprehensive review.[4] Appropriate antimicrobials for initial therapy and that can be used as suppression are listed in **Table 1**.[9] Selected situations, however, that may either be frequently encountered in clinical practice or are particularly challenging are discussed later.

Staphylococcal Infection Treated with Débridement, Antibiotics, and Implant Retention

Staphylococci are the most frequent cause of PJI overall.[4] When treated as part of a TSE procedure and after resection, definitive monotherapy is typically with vancomycin or a parenteral β-lactam for MRSA or MSSA, respectively. For staphylo-coccal infection treated with DAIR, multiple studies have demonstrated a greater likeli-hood of success when rifampin is combined with a companion antibiotic, compared with pathogen-directed monotherapy.[55,69–71] Oral rifampin is most often given with a parenteral agent for the first 2 weeks to 6 weeks, followed by a quinolone or other oral companion medication with rifampin to complete 3 months to 6 months. Histori-cally, a 6-month course of rifampin-based therapy has been used for knee infection, whereas a 3-month course is used for other joints.[9] Rifampin-based combination ther-apy is also appropriate when using the OSE procedure. The use of rifampin presents specific challenges with regard to drug-drug interactions and must be carefully moni-tored, both at the time of rifampin initiation and more importantly at the time of discon-tinuation. After completion of rifampin-combination therapy, suppression is typically used for at least some period of time. The need for indefinite suppression in this situ-ation is highly controversial.[9] Fluoroquinolone monotherapy should not be used for suppression due to the risk of emergent resistance.[69] An outline of the use of rifampin for PJI is shown in **Fig. 1**.

Culture-Negative Prosthetic Joint Infection

Reasons for culture-negative PJI include preceding antimicrobial therapy,[72] insuffi-cient use of available tools to identify a known pathogen, infection with a pathogen that cannot be identified using available methods,[73] or a noninfectious mimic of PJI.[74] A majority of patients with culture-negative PJI have received recent antimicro-bial therapy.[75] The antimicrobial treatment plan should be designed to incorporate the spectrum of the preceding antimicrobial(s), along with the known microbiology of PJI according to the joint, time period, and host.[4] Few data suggest that TSE may be the strategy of choice,[75] possibly due to the local antimicrobial therapy provided by the ALC, but only prospective studies will answer this question definitively.

Fungal Prosthetic Joint Infection

Although a cause of less than 1% of PJI,[4] fungi are often difficult to treat when encoun-tered. *Candida* species are the most common cause of fungal PJI and are typically found in the setting of prior arthroplasty revision and/or prior PJI.[76,77] Antimicrobial treatment of fungal osteoarticular infection is typically prolonged[78] and the available literature support the use of TSE or resection-based strategy rather than implant retention.[77,79]

Nonsurgical Prosthetic Joint Infection Management

Antimicrobial therapy without accompanying surgery most often results in a delay in appropriate management and confusion regarding the microbiologic diagnosis. Accordingly, nonsurgical management is not recommended. It may be considered, however, for those who are unable to undergo even a single surgical procedure, when accompanied by appropriate counseling. Infection with microorganisms that are susceptible to oral antibiotics is a prerequisite for this consideration. A nonsurgical strategy is likely to be more successful in those with early rather than delayed or chronic infection.[80] Typically, nonsurgical treatment is attempted with joint aspiration to determine the microbiology of infection, followed by 4 weeks to 6 weeks of pathogen-directed intravenous or highly bioavailable oral antimicrobials. Many pa-tients ultimately are placed on prolonged or indefinite oral antimicrobial suppression.

SUMMARY

Although challenging to cure, PJI may be successfully managed through a collaborative relationship between infectious diseases physicians and orthopedic surgeons. Accurate microbiologic diagnosis, a careful selection of a medical/surgical strategy, and anticipation and management of encountered complications may yield a successful outcome for each patient. Future studies should continue to define the ideal medical/surgical strategy for each type of infection, whether oral or parenteral therapy is needed for each strategy, and what the role is for antimicrobial suppression. Ultimately, the development of large, multi-institutional networks may be necessary to ask and answer these remaining difficult questions.

REFERENCES

1. Diaz-Ledezma C, Higuera CA, Parvizi J. Success after treatment of periprosthetic joint infection: a Delphi-based international multidisciplinary consensus. Clin Orthop 2013;471(7):2374–82.
2. Tsaras G, Osmon DR, Mabry T, et al. Incidence, secular trends, and outcomes of prosthetic joint infection: a population-based study, Olmsted county, Minnesota, 1969-2007. Infect Control Hosp Epidemiol 2012;33(12):1207–12.
3. Key JA. Sulfonamides in the treatment of chronic osteomyelitis. J Bone Joint Surg Am 1944;26(1):63–70.
4. Tande AJ, Patel R. Prosthetic joint infection. Clin Microbiol Rev 2014;27(2): 302–45.
5. Tice AD, Rehm SJ, Dalovisio JR, et al. Practice guidelines for outpatient parenteral antimicrobial therapy. IDSA guidelines. Clin Infect Dis 2004;38(12):1651–72.
6. Hanada Y, Berbari EF, Steckelberg JM. Minocycline-induced cutaneous hyperpigmentation in an orthopedic patient population. Open Forum Infect Dis 2016; 3(1):ofv107.
7. Moran E, Byren I, Atkins BL. The diagnosis and management of prosthetic joint infections. J Antimicrob Chemother 2010;65(Suppl 3):iii45–54.
8. Leone S, Borre S, Monforte A, et al. Consensus document on controversial issues in the diagnosis and treatment of prosthetic joint infections. Int J Infect Dis 2010; 14(Suppl 4):S67–77.
9. Osmon DR, Berbari EF, Berendt AR, et al. Diagnosis and management of prosthetic joint infection: clinical practice guidelines by the Infectious Diseases Society of America. Clin Infect Dis 2013;56(1):e1–25.
10. Zimmerli W, Trampuz A, Ochsner PE. Prosthetic-joint infections. N Engl J Med 2004;351(16):1645–54.
11. De Man FH, Sendi P, Zimmerli W, et al. Infectiological, functional, and radiographic outcome after revision for prosthetic hip infection according to a strict algorithm. Acta Orthop 2011;82(1):27–34.
12. Betsch BY, Eggli S, Siebenrock KA, et al. Treatment of joint prosthesis infection in accordance with current recommendations improves outcome. Clin Infect Dis 2008;46(8):1221–6.
13. Giulieri SG, Graber P, Ochsner PE, et al. Management of infection associated with total hip arthroplasty according to a treatment algorithm. Infection 2004;32(4): 222–8.
14. Rand JA, Bryan RS. Reimplantation for the salvage of an infected total knee arthroplasty. J Bone Joint Surg Am 1983;65(8):1081–6.
15. Mont MA, Waldman BJ, Hungerford DS. Evaluation of preoperative cultures before second-stage reimplantation of a total knee prosthesis complicated by

infection. A comparison-group study. J Bone Joint Surg Am 2000;82-A(11): 1552–7.

16. Kusuma SK, Ward J, Jacofsky M, et al. What is the role of serological testing between stages of two-stage reconstruction of the infected prosthetic knee? Clin Orthop Relat Res 2011;469(4):1002–8.

17. Ghanem E, Azzam K, Seeley M, et al. Staged revision for knee arthroplasty infection: what is the role of serologic tests before reimplantation? Clin Orthop Relat Res 2009;467(7):1699–705.

18. Frangiamore SJ, Siqueira MB, Saleh A, et al. Synovial Cytokines and the MSIS criteria are not useful for determining infection resolution after periprosthetic joint infection explantation. Clin Orthop Relat Res 2016;474(7):1630–9.

19. George J, Kwiecien G, Klika AK, et al. Are frozen sections and MSIS criteria reliable at the time of reimplantation of two-stage revision arthroplasty? Clin Orthop Relat Res 2016;474(7):1619–26.

20. Masri BA, Duncan CP, Beauchamp CP. Long-term elution of antibiotics from bone-cement: an in vivo study using the prosthesis of antibiotic-loaded acrylic cement (PROSTALAC) system. J Arthroplasty 1998;13(3):331–8.

21. Sterling GJ, Crawford S, Potter JH, et al. The pharmacokinetics of Simplex-tobramycin bone cement. J Bone Joint Surg Br 2003;85(5):646–9.

22. Iarikov D, Demian H, Rubin D, et al. Choice and doses of antibacterial agents for cement spacers in treatment of prosthetic joint infections: review of published studies. Clin Infect Dis 2012;55(11):1474–80.

23. Silvestre A, Almeida F, Renovell P, et al. Revision of infected total knee arthroplasty: two-stage reimplantation using an antibiotic-impregnated static spacer. Clin Orthop Surg 2013;5(3):180–7.

24. McKenna PB, O'Shea K, Masterson EL. Two-stage revision of infected hip arthroplasty using a shortened post-operative course of antibiotics. Arch Orthop Trauma Surg 2009;129(4):489–94.

25. Stockley I, Mockford BJ, Hoad-Reddick A, et al. The use of two-stage exchange arthroplasty with depot antibiotics in the absence of long-term antibiotic therapy in infected total hip replacement. J Bone Joint Surg Br 2008;90(2):145–8.

26. Frank JM, Kayupov E, Moric M, et al. The Mark Coventry, MD, award: oral antibiotics reduce reinfection after two-stage exchange: a multicenter, randomized controlled trial. Clin Orthop Relat Res 2017;475(1):56–61.

27. Zywiel MG, Johnson AJ, Stroh DA, et al. Prophylactic oral antibiotics reduce reinfection rates following two-stage revision total knee arthroplasty. Int Orthop 2011; 35(1):37–42.

28. Lange J, Troelsen A, Thomsen RW, et al. Chronic infections in hip arthroplasties: comparing risk of reinfection following one-stage and two-stage revision: a systematic review and meta-analysis. Clin Epidemiol 2012;4:57–73.

29. Jamsen E, Stogiannidis I, Malmivaara A, et al. Outcome of prosthesis exchange for infected knee arthroplasty: the effect of treatment approach. Acta Orthop 2009;80(1):67–77.

30. Biring GS, Kostamo T, Garbuz DS, et al. Two-stage revision arthroplasty of the hip for infection using an interim articulated Prostalac hip spacer: a 10- to 15-year follow-up study. J Bone Joint Surg Br 2009;91(11):1431–7.

31. Nelson GN, Davis DE, Namdari S. Outcomes in the treatment of periprosthetic joint infection after shoulder arthroplasty: a systematic review. J Shoulder Elbow Surg 2016;25(8):1337–45.

32. Cheung EV, Adams RA, Morrey BF. Reimplantation of a total elbow prosthesis following resection arthroplasty for infection. J Bone Joint Surg Am 2008;90(3): 589–94.

33. Kubista B, Hartzler RU, Wood CM, et al. Reinfection after two-stage revision for periprosthetic infection of total knee arthroplasty. Int Orthop 2012;36(1):65–71.

34. Mortazavi SM, Vegari D, Ho A, et al. Two-stage exchange arthroplasty for infected total knee arthroplasty: predictors of failure. Clin Orthop 2011;469(11):3049–54.

35. Bejon P, Berendt A, Atkins BL, et al. Two-stage revision for prosthetic joint infection: predictors of outcome and the role of reimplantation microbiology. J Antimicrob Chemother 2010;65(3):569–75.

36. Hirakawa K, Stulberg BN, Wilde AH, et al. Results of 2-stage reimplantation for infected total knee arthroplasty. J Arthroplasty 1998;13(1):22–8.

37. Hsieh PH, Huang KC, Shih HN. Prosthetic joint infection in patients with rheumatoid arthritis: an outcome analysis compared with controls. PLoS One 2013;8(8): e71666.

38. Hanssen AD, Rand JA, Osmon DR. Treatment of the infected total knee arthroplasty with insertion of another prosthesis. The effect of antibiotic-impregnated bone cement. Clin Orthop 1994;309(309):44–55.

39. Zmistowski B, Tetreault MW, Alijanipour P, et al. Recurrent periprosthetic joint infection: persistent or new infection? J Arthroplasty 2013;28(9):1486–9.

40. Namba RS, Inacio MC, Paxton EW. Risk factors associated with deep surgical site infections after primary total knee arthroplasty: an analysis of 56,216 knees. J Bone Joint Surg Am 2013;95(9):775–82.

41. Peersman G, Laskin R, Davis J, et al. Infection in total knee replacement: a retrospective review of 6489 total knee replacements. Clin Orthop 2001;(392):15–23.

42. Namba RS, Inacio MC, Paxton EW. Risk factors associated with surgical site infection in 30,491 primary total hip replacements. J Bone Joint Surg Br 2012; 94(10):1330–8.

43. Berbari EF, Osmon DR, Lahr B, et al. The Mayo prosthetic joint infection risk score: implication for surgical site infection reporting and risk stratification. Infect Control Hosp Epidemiol 2012;33(8):774–81.

44. Rudelli S, Uip D, Honda E, et al. One-stage revision of infected total hip arthroplasty with bone graft. J Arthroplasty 2008;23(8):1165–77.

45. Whiteside LA, Peppers M, Nayfeh TA, et al. Methicillin-resistant Staphylococcus aureus in TKA treated with revision and direct intra-articular antibiotic infusion. Clin Orthop 2011;469(1):26–33.

46. Raut VV, Siney PD, Wroblewski BM. One-stage revision of infected total hip replacements with discharging sinuses. J Bone Joint Surg Br 1994;76(5):721–4.

47. Wroblewski BM. One-stage revision of infected cemented total hip arthroplasty. Clin Orthop 1986;(211):103–7.

48. Callaghan JJ, Katz RP, Johnston RC. One-stage revision surgery of the infected hip. A minimum 10-year followup study. Clin Orthop 1999;369(369):139–43.

49. Ince A, Seemann K, Frommelt L, et al. One-stage exchange shoulder arthroplasty for peri-prosthetic infection. J Bone Joint Surg Br 2005;87(6):814–8.

50. Silva M, Tharani R, Schmalzried TP. Results of direct exchange or debridement of the infected total knee arthroplasty. Clin Orthop 2002;404(404):125–31.

51. Brandt CM, Sistrunk WW, Duffy MC, et al. Staphylococcus aureus prosthetic joint infection treated with debridement and prosthesis retention. Clin Infect Dis 1997; 24(5):914–9.

52. Byren I, Bejon P, Atkins BL, et al. One hundred and twelve infected arthroplasties treated with 'DAIR' (debridement, antibiotics and implant retention): antibiotic duration and outcome. J Antimicrob Chemother 2009;63(6):1264–71.
53. Marculescu CE, Berbari EF, Hanssen AD, et al. Outcome of prosthetic joint infections treated with debridement and retention of components. Clin Infect Dis 2006; 42(4):471–8.
54. Rodriguez-Pardo D, Pigrau C, Lora-Tamayo J, et al. Gram-negative prosthetic joint infection: outcome of a debridement, antibiotics and implant retention approach. A large multicentre study. Clin Microbiol Infect 2014;20(11):O911–9.
55. Lora-Tamayo J, Murillo O, Iribarren JA, et al. A large multicenter study of methicillin-susceptible and methicillin-resistant Staphylococcus aureus prosthetic joint infections managed with implant retention. Clin Infect Dis 2013; 56(2):182–94.
56. Konigsberg BS, Valle CJ, Ting NT, et al. Acute hematogenous infection following total hip and knee arthroplasty. J Arthroplasty 2013;29(3):469–72.
57. Koyonos L, Zmistowski B, Della Valle CJ, et al. Infection control rate of irrigation and debridement for periprosthetic joint infection. Clin Orthop 2011;469(11): 3043–8.
58. Azzam KA, Seeley M, Ghanem E, et al. Irrigation and debridement in the management of prosthetic joint infection: traditional indications revisited. J Arthroplasty 2010;25(7):1022–7.
59. Soriano A, Garcia S, Bori G, et al. Treatment of acute post-surgical infection of joint arthroplasty. Clin Microbiol Infect 2006;12(9):930–3.
60. Jaen N, Martinez-Pastor JC, Munoz-Mahamud E, et al. Long-term outcome of acute prosthetic joint infections due to gram-negative bacilli treated with retention of prosthesis. Rev Esp Quimioter 2012;25(3):194–8.
61. Crockarell JR, Hanssen AD, Osmon DR, et al. Treatment of infection with debridement and retention of the components following hip arthroplasty. J Bone Joint Surg Am 1998;80(9):1306–13.
62. Barberan J, Aguilar L, Carroquino G, et al. Conservative treatment of staphylococcal prosthetic joint infections in elderly patients. Am J Med 2006;119(11): 993.e7-10.
63. Castellanos J, Flores X, Llusa M, et al. The Girdlestone pseudarthrosis in the treatment of infected hip replacements. Int Orthop 1998;22(3):178–81.
64. Choi HR, Freiberg AA, Malchau H, et al. The fate of unplanned retention of prosthetic articulating spacers for infected total hip and total knee arthroplasty. J Arthroplasty 2014;29(4):690–3.
65. Mabry TM, Jacofsky DJ, Haidukewych GJ, et al. Comparison of intramedullary nailing and external fixation knee arthrodesis for the infected knee replacement. Clin Orthop 2007;464:11–5.
66. Sierra RJ, Trousdale RT, Pagnano MW. Above-the-knee amputation after a total knee replacement: prevalence, etiology, and functional outcome. J Bone Joint Surg Am 2003;85-A(6):1000–4.
67. Steckel H, Baums MH, Tennstedt-Schenk C, et al. Necrotizing fasciitis of the knee following primary total knee arthroplasty. Knee Surg Sports Traumatol Arthrosc 2011;19(12):2076–9.
68. Fedorka CJ, Chen AF, McGarry WM, et al. Functional ability after above-the-knee amputation for infected total knee arthroplasty. Clin Orthop 2011;469(4):1024–32.
69. Zimmerli W, Widmer AF, Blatter M, et al. Role of rifampin for treatment of orthopedic implant-related staphylococcal infections: a randomized controlled trial. Foreign-Body Infection (FBI) Study Group. JAMA 1998;279(19):1537–41.

70. El Helou OC, Berbari EF, Lahr BD, et al. Efficacy and safety of rifampin containing regimen for staphylococcal prosthetic joint infections treated with debridement and retention. Eur J Clin Microbiol Infect Dis 2010;29(8):961–7.
71. Senneville E, Joulie D, Legout L, et al. Outcome and predictors of treatment failure in total hip/knee prosthetic joint infections due to Staphylococcus aureus. Clin Infect Dis 2011;53(4):334–40.
72. Malekzadeh D, Osmon DR, Lahr BD, et al. Prior use of antimicrobial therapy is a risk factor for culture-negative prosthetic joint infection. Clin Orthop Relat Res 2010;468(8):2039–45.
73. Tande AJ, Cunningham SA, Raoult D, et al. A case of Q fever prosthetic joint infection and description of an assay for detection of Coxiella burnetii. J Clin Microbiol 2013;51(1):66–9.
74. Mikhael MM, Hanssen AD, Sierra RJ. Failure of metal-on-metal total hip arthroplasty mimicking hip infection. A report of two cases. J Bone Joint Surg Am 2009;91(2):443–6.
75. Berbari EF, Marculescu C, Sia I, et al. Culture-negative prosthetic joint infection. Clin Infect Dis 2007;45(9):1113–9.
76. Hwang BH, Yoon JY, Nam CH, et al. Fungal peri-prosthetic joint infection after primary total knee replacement. J Bone Joint Surg Br 2012;94(5):656–9.
77. Azzam K, Parvizi J, Jungkind D, et al. Microbiological, clinical, and surgical features of fungal prosthetic joint infections: a multi-institutional experience. J Bone Joint Surg Am 2009;91(Suppl 6):142–9.
78. Pappas PG, Kauffman CA, Andes DR, et al. Clinical practice guideline for the management of candidiasis: 2016 Update by the Infectious Diseases Society of America. Clin Infect Dis 2016;62(4):e1–50.
79. Kuiper JW, van den Bekerom MP, van der Stappen J, et al. 2-stage revision recommended for treatment of fungal hip and knee prosthetic joint infections. Acta Orthop 2013;84(6):517–23.
80. Pavoni GL, Giannella M, Falcone M, et al. Conservative medical therapy of prosthetic joint infections: retrospective analysis of an 8-year experience. Clin Microbiol Infect 2004;10(9):831–7.

Prevention of Infection in Orthopedic Prosthetic Surgery

Ioana Chirca, MD[a], Camelia Marculescu, MD, MSCR[b],*

KEYWORDS

- Orthopedic • Infection • Prosthetic joint • Prophylaxis

KEY POINTS

- Prosthetic joint surgery is the last resort in the treatment of osteoarthritis and other degenerative joint diseases and is sometimes complicated by infection.
- Prevention of infection in total joint arthroplasty is a multidisciplinary approach and involves patient-related and procedure-related factors along with postoperative care.
- Some prevention strategies are still controversial, and more research is needed; research of innovative materials and approaches to prevent infection is underway.

INTRODUCTION

Orthopedic prosthetic surgery has become a fairly frequent and safe orthopedic procedure. Data from the National Center for Health Statistics show only in 2010 more than a million total hip replacements and knee replacements were performed. It is estimated that approximately 4 million patients will benefit from a total joint replacement by 2030.[1] Postoperative prosthetic joint infections (PJI) are a rare (<2%)[2,3] but significant complication, with high functional, psychosocial, financial, and economic impact on the patients and the health care system. In the current environment, it is projected that the cost of caring for the infected orthopedic implants will exceed 1.62 billion dollars by 2020.[4]

Recently, a standardized definition of PJI was established, and several classifications are available, with respect to the timing of the clinical manifestations (early, delayed, late, and silent) and pathogenesis (exogenous or hematogenous).[5,6] The most common causative organisms are *Staphylococcus aureus* (SA), coagulase-negative staphylococci, and streptococci, which constitute skin flora, and underscore the exogenous route as the most frequent mechanism of infection.[7] The hematogenous

Disclosure Statement: The authors have nothing to disclose.
[a] Department of infectious Diseases, University Hospital, 1350 Walton Way, Augusta, GA 30909, USA; [b] Division of Infectious Diseases, Medical University of South Carolina, 171 Ashley Avenue, Charleston, SC 29425, USA
* Corresponding author.
E-mail address: marcule@musc.edu

Infect Dis Clin N Am 31 (2017) 253–263
http://dx.doi.org/10.1016/j.idc.2017.01.011
0891-5520/17/Published by Elsevier Inc.

id.theclinics.com

seeding of prosthesis from distant sites is mostly a late complication and represents a significant risk for organisms such as SA.[8] In addition, the fine balance between the individual patient factors, local prosthetic factors, organism virulence, and inoculum size dictates the development of a PJI. Hence, the prevention of PJI is a matter of perioperative optimization of the patient, careful preoperative, intraoperative, and postoperative measures to prevent infection.

Risk Factors

Several factors are involved in the development of a PJI, and they pertain to individual, patient-related factors as well as procedural and postprocedural factors, some clearly demonstrated in studies, others with a somewhat looser association (**Table 1**). Attempts were made to create composite risk scores to assist in the preoperative evaluation. The National Nosocomial Infections Surveillance score, for example, includes the length of procedure, the American Society of Anesthesiologists (ASA) score, and the surgical wound classification.[9]

PREOPERATIVE FACTORS

The preoperative risk factors mostly pertain to patient optimization and require a multidisciplinary approach, ideally with the involvement of the primary care physician, endocrinologist, and rheumatologist if necessary.

Obesity and Malnutrition

Obesity, malnutrition, and obesity with malnutrition were found to be associated with an increased risk of PJI in multiple studies.[10–13] Malnutrition is associated with impaired wound healing and immunity, hence an increased risk of infection. Although the association of poor nutritional status with increased risk for PJI is well established, there is

Table 1		
Risk factors associated with development of prosthetic joint infection		
Preoperative (Patient) Factors	**Perioperative and Intraoperative Factors**	**Postoperative Factors**
Obesity (body mass index >35)[12,13,22,70]	Prolonged duration of procedure[9,22]	Hematoma[9,22]
Malnutrition[10]	Antimicrobial prophylaxis[42,43]	Superficial surgical site infection[9]
Smoking[20,71]	Revision vs primary arthroplasty[72]	Wound drainage/dehiscence[9,22]
Anemia[23]	Metal-to-metal vs metal-to-plastic prosthesis[72,73]	Allogeneic blood transfusion[22]
DM[12]	Simultaneous bilateral procedure[22]	Acute coronary event or atrial fibrillation[22]
Inflammatory arthropathies[9,24]	Cement without antibiotic[72,74]	Perioperative infections at a distant site[22]
Malignancy[75]	Operating room (OR) traffic[60–62]	Invasive procedures with high bacteremic risk[64–66]
Immunosuppressive medication[25,26]	Laminar airflow in the OR[58,59]	
ASA >2[22]	Equipment contamination[76]	
SA colonization status[33,34,77]	Hypothermia[78,79]	
Antecedent septic arthritis[9]	Hair clipping[80]	
Genetic susceptibility[81]	Skin preparation and draping[82,83]	

no study to date to demonstrate an improvement of PJI rates with correction of malnutrition. An albumin level less than 3.5 g/dL, leukocyte count less than 1500 cells/mm^3, and transferrin level less than 200 mg/dL are widely considered serum markers for malnutrition, and they should be evaluated and optimized preoperatively. It is perhaps more practical to correct malnutrition than obesity, especially in these patients with poor functional status and reduced exercise capacity due to joint disease.

Perioperative Hyperglycemia and Diabetes Control

Diabetes mellitus (DM) and preoperative and postoperative hyperglycemia were found to be more prevalent in patients who develop PJI in one study, with postoperative blood sugar levels greater than 200 mg/dL being found to increase the risk of infection by 2-fold.[14] Another study shows that patients with uncontrolled DM were at higher risk to develop postoperative complications after total joint arthroplasty (TJA), including infection.[15] Recently, it was found that perioperative hyperglycemia is common (40%) in TJA patients, and pre-existent DM is the strongest risk factor for the development of severe hyperglycemia; preoperative increased levels of glycosylated hemoglobin and fasting glucose were associated with development of perioperative hyperglycemia.[16] Therefore, patients with known DM should be well controlled preoperatively, with hemoglobin A1c (HbA$_{1C}$) as close as possible to normal and all patients screened preoperatively with an HbA$_{1C}$ or at least a fasting blood glucose level. A perioperative blood sugar level of 80 to 180 mg/dL is currently recommended.[17] Although the optimal HbA$_{1C}$ level at which TJA risks become excessive has not been established, the International Consensus Meeting statement recommends preoperative optimization of blood glucose and would only very carefully consider offering elective arthroplasty to patients in whom the fasting glucose level is greater than 200 mg/dL (10 mmol/L) and HbA$_{1C}$ >7%.[18,19]

Smoking

Current and past smoking increase the risk of PJI significantly, probably related to local vasoconstriction in the surgical bed with subsequent impaired wound healing. It is recommended the patients should abstain from tobacco use at least 4 weeks preoperatively.[20,21]

Anemia

Pre-existent anemia increases the risk of PJI, although it has not been shown yet that preoperative correction of this will decrease PJI rates. More patients with preoperative anemia require postoperative blood transfusions, which have also been shown to increase the risk for PJI.[22,23] Given these data, correction of preoperative anemia with iron and perhaps erythropoietin may decrease the need of transfusion and subsequently the PJI risk.

Rheumatoid Arthritis and Immunosuppressive Medications

Patients with rheumatoid arthritis often require a TJA. Several studies have shown an increased risk of developing PJI for these patients, partly because of their unique immune makeup, partly because of the immunosuppressive medications.[9,24–26] The available data are mostly equivocal, with conflicting results.[25,27] The American College of Rheumatology recommendation is to withhold tumor necrosis alpha inhibitors around the time of elective surgery for the duration of time equaling 3 to 5 times half-life of the drug if stopping the drug is thought beneficial. For methotrexate, the general approach is to stop the treatment the week before the surgery.[28–30] These medications should be generally restarted after the surgical site healing occurs

(2–4 weeks). However, these recommendations are based on equivocal data, and they should be individualized.

Staphylococcus aureus Screening and Decolonization

SA is a major cause of PJI, along with coagulase-negative staphylococci.[30–32] The major site of colonization is the anterior nares, but it was found that SA was concomitantly discovered at other body sites such as axilla and inguinal. One study found that preoperative screening for SA and nasal decolonization with mupirocin is effective at not only eradicating SA but also decreasing by 5 times endogenous SA infections in orthopedic prosthetic surgery.[33] Hacek and colleagues[34] demonstrated a 4-fold decrease in the rates of SA surgical site infection following TJA with a program of screening and 5-day mupirocin decolonization. Decolonization at other body sites by using an at-home protocol with chlorhexidine (CHG) the night before and morning of surgery was proved effective in some studies and had no effect in others for orthopedic surgery.[35–37] Use of both nasal mupirocin and CHG proved effective at preventing surgical site infection, inclusive of orthopedic infections, in hospitalized patients colonized with SA.[38] The general recommendation is for a combined approach for preoperative screening followed by decolonization with mupirocin for 5 days preoperatively and CHG use the night before and the morning of surgery.[21,39] Despite the wide acceptance and implementation of the preoperative decolonization protocol, new data emerged recently showing persistence of colonization in 20% to 30% of the patients.[40,41] The clinical significance of this data is to be investigated, but concerns about emergence of mupirocin-resistant SA as well as cost-related issues have led to research of alternative agents to replace mupirocin (povidone-iodine, Retapamulin).

INTRAOPERATIVE FACTORS
Perioperative Antimicrobial Prophylaxis

Current data support the use of perioperative antimicrobial prophylaxis (PAP) as the most effective strategy to prevent surgical site infections in general and PJI in particular.[42,43] The recommendations for antimicrobial selection, the timing of administration, dosing regimen, and intraoperative redosing are summarized in **Table 2**.[39]

The preferred preoperative antibiotic in TJA is cefazolin (or cefuroxime) unless there is known MRSA colonization status or the patient has a type I allergic reaction to beta-lactams. In that case, clindamycin and vancomycin are the preferred agents. Although some studies suggest an advantage of vancomycin in preventing surgical site infections in high-prevalence settings, others have not shown any clear benefit of vancomycin over beta-lactams.[42,44–46] At this time, vancomycin cannot be recommended routinely in non–methicillin-resistant *Staphylococcus aureus* (MRSA) colonized patients

Table 2				
Recommendations for perioperative antimicrobial prophylaxis				
Antimicrobial Agent	Indication	Dose	Half-Life (for Normal Creatinine Clearance)	Intraoperative Redosing Interval
Cefazolin	Not MRSA colonized	2 g (3 g for obese or >120 kg)	1.2–2.2 h	4 h
Clindamycin	Allergy to penicillin	900 mg	2–4 h	6 h
Vancomycin	MRSA colonized and/or allergy to penicillin	15 mg/kg	4–8 h	Not indicated

because it has known lower efficacy than beta-lactams against methicillin-susceptible SA, longer infusion time, and little supportive data. The addition of vancomycin to cefazolin did not appear to decrease the rate of surgical site infections, but decreased the incidence of MRSA infection, with a high number needed to treat.[47] Current guidelines recommend the use of vancomycin only in institutions with known high rates of MRSA surgical site infections and in patients with known MRSA colonization.[39]

Apart from antimicrobial selection, careful consideration must be given to dose, timing of the dose, redosing, and duration, because these factors have a high impact in the efficacy of the antimicrobial prophylaxis.

- Dose: Some experts recommend an increase of cefazolin dose in obese patients to 3 g, based on pharmacokinetic data and expert opinion; some clinical data available at this time do not support such dosing adjustment in this setting.[48,49] Vancomycin should be dosed at 15 to 20 mg/kg of actual body weight, because there is high variability in tissue penetration in obesity.[50]
- Timing: Cefazolin should be given within 30 to 60 minutes before surgical incision. Vancomycin should be started 60 to 120 minutes before the incision and continued intraoperatively if needed.
- Redosing: Cefazolin has a short half-life (1.2–2.2 hours); hence, the need for a repeat dose if procedures exceed 4 hours or if there is significant blood loss of over 2000 mL. Clindamycin has a half-life of 4 hours and rarely requires intraoperative redosing for procedures longer than 6 hours. Vancomycin does not require a second dose due to the long half-life.
- Duration: The current guidelines do not support PAP beyond 24 hours. One randomized trial did not demonstrate any difference in surgical site infections in orthopedic surgery procedures for 24 hours versus 7 days of PAP.[51]

Antibiotic-Impregnated Bone Cement and Antibiotic-Laden Implants

Addition of antibiotic to the bone cement was shown to lower the PJI rates by 50% for primary hip arthroplasties and by 40% in revisions of previously infected hips.[52] Another meta-analysis showed a benefit in using antibiotic-impregnated bone cement in prevention of deep infection for primary TJA.[53] In a prospective Dutch study,[54] antibiotic-impregnated cement did not prevent surgical infections in total hip arthroplasties. Currently, antibiotic-impregnated cement is approved in the United States for prophylaxis in the second stage of a 2-stage revision arthroplasty following an infection but not for prophylaxis of infection in primary TJA.[39] The International Consensus Meeting guidelines advise limiting the use of antibiotic-impregnated cement during elective primary arthroplasty to patients at high risk of PJI (such as those with diabetes or immunosuppressive conditions).[18,19] Antibiotic, silver-coated, and adhesion-resistant implants are still in research, but the in vitro studies are promising.[55]

Skin Preparation and Draping

- Several skin antiseptics are available, the most common ones being alcohol-based CHG preparations and povidone-iodine. A recent meta-analysis found some evidence that alcohol-based CHG has an advantage in preventing surgical infections in clean surgeries compared with iodine.[56] However, the same meta-analysis suggests there is insufficient evidence to recommend one or the other. Other considerations such as cost and availability should be considered when choosing the skin antiseptic.
- A *Cochrane Review* from 2015 found no evidence that adhesive drapes offer any advantage in preventing surgical infections compared with nonadhesive ones.[57]

Operating Room Traffic and Laminar Flow

- Laminar airflow, although theoretically advantageous, has not had convincing evidence to support its use since introduction in the 1960s.[58,59]
- Multiple studies have shown that reducing traffic in the operating room would decrease operating room air bacterial counts and that there are multiple opportunities to reduce the traffic and subsequently the rate of surgical site infections.[60–62]

POSTOPERATIVE FACTORS
Infection at Distant Sites and Preprocedure Prophylaxis

Postoperative bacteremia, especially early after surgery, has been shown to increase the risk of prosthetic seeding and infection.[8] Postoperative bacteremia should be promptly recognized and treated. Although asymptomatic bacteriuria has been identified as a risk factor for PJI, antibiotic treatment did not elicit a benefit.[63] Postoperative urinary tract infections, respiratory infections, and other infections with bacteremic potential should be recognized and treated promptly.

Antibiotic prophylaxis before dental procedures has been routinely recommended for many years, but recent evidence does not support this practice.[64,65] Currently, good oral hygiene is encouraged rather than antimicrobial prophylaxis before dental procedures.

So far, neither urologic nor gastroenterologic procedures have been associated with an increased risk for development of a PJI, with the exception of a single-center, case-control study that found an increased risk associated with esophagogastroduodenoscopy with biopsy.[66,67] No recommendation for antibiotic prophylaxis has been made based on the current evidence.

Hematoma Formation and Wound Drainage

Hematoma formation and persistent wound drainage have been found to increase the risk for PJI so careful monitoring and early intervention may mitigate some adverse outcomes.[9,22,68] Aggressive anticoagulation postoperatively is associated with hematoma formation and is discouraged. Early intervention on draining wounds has proved beneficial.[69]

SUMMARY

Prevention of PJI requires a multifaceted approach and a dedicated team. It involves preoperative medical optimization of the patient, careful surgical technique, appropriate antimicrobial selection for prophylaxis, and postoperative monitoring of the surgical site for early recognition of complications.

REFERENCES

1. Kurtz S, Ong K, Lau E, et al. Projections of primary and revision hip and knee arthroplasty in the United States from 2005 to 2030. J Bone Joint Surg Am 2007;89: 780–5.
2. Edwards JR, Peterson KD, Mu Y, et al. National Healthcare Safety Network (NHSN) report: data summary for 2006 through 2008, issued December 2009. Am J Infect Control 2009;37:783–805.
3. Rosenthal VD, Richtmann R, Singh S, et al. Surgical site infections, International Nosocomial Infection Control Consortium (INICC) report, data summary of 30 countries, 2005-2010. Infect Control Hosp Epidemiol 2013;34:597–604.

4. Kurtz SM, Lau E, Watson H, et al. Economic burden of periprosthetic joint infection in the United States. J Arthroplasty 2012;27:61–5.e1.
5. Parvizi J, Zmistowski B, Berbari EF, et al. New definition for periprosthetic joint infection: from the workgroup of the Musculoskeletal Infection Society. Clin Orthop Relat Res 2011;469:2992–4.
6. Zimmerli W, Trampuz A, Ochsner PE. Prosthetic-joint infections. N Engl J Med 2004;351:1645–54.
7. Tsukayama DT, Estrada R, Gustilo RB. Infection after total hip arthroplasty. A study of the treatment of one hundred and six infections. J Bone Joint Surg Am 1996;78:512–23.
8. Murdoch DR, Roberts SA, Fowler VG Jr, et al. Infection of orthopedic prostheses after Staphylococcus aureus bacteremia. Clin Infect Dis 2001;32:647–9.
9. Berbari EF, Hanssen AD, Duffy MC, et al. Risk factors for prosthetic joint infection: case-control study. Clin Infect Dis 1998;27:1247–54.
10. Yi PH, Frank RM, Vann E, et al. Is potential malnutrition associated with septic failure and acute infection after revision total joint arthroplasty? Clin Orthop Relat Res 2015;473:175–82.
11. Peersman G, Laskin R, Davis J, et al. Infection in total knee replacement: a retrospective review of 6489 total knee replacements. Clin Orthop Relat Res 2001;(392): 15–23.
12. Jamsen E, Nevalainen P, Eskelinen A, et al. Obesity, diabetes, and preoperative hyperglycemia as predictors of periprosthetic joint infection: a single-center analysis of 7181 primary hip and knee replacements for osteoarthritis. J Bone Joint Surg Am 2012;94:e101.
13. Kerkhoffs GM, Servien E, Dunn W, et al. The influence of obesity on the complication rate and outcome of total knee arthroplasty: a meta-analysis and systematic literature review. J Bone Joint Surg Am 2012;94:1839–44.
14. Mraovic B, Suh D, Jacovides C, et al. Perioperative hyperglycemia and postoperative infection after lower limb arthroplasty. J Diabetes Sci Technol 2011;5: 412–8.
15. Marchant MH Jr, Viens NA, Cook C, et al. The impact of glycemic control and diabetes mellitus on perioperative outcomes after total joint arthroplasty. J Bone Joint Surg Am 2009;91:1621–9.
16. Jamsen E, Nevalainen PI, Eskelinen A, et al. Risk factors for perioperative hyperglycemia in primary hip and knee replacements. Acta Orthop 2015;86:175–82.
17. Standards of medical care in diabetes—2016: summary of revisions. Diabetes Care 2016;39(Suppl 1):S4–5.
18. Parvizi J, Gehrke T. International consensus on periprosthetic joint infection: let cumulative wisdom be a guide. J Bone Joint Surg Am 2014;96:441.
19. Parvizi J, Gehrke T, Chen AF. Proceedings of the International Consensus on Periprosthetic Joint Infection. Bone Joint J 2013;95-B:1450–2.
20. Singh JA. Smoking and outcomes after knee and hip arthroplasty: a systematic review. J Rheumatol 2011;38:1824–34.
21. Alexander JW, Solomkin JS, Edwards MJ. Updated recommendations for control of surgical site infections. Ann Surg 2011;253:1082–93.
22. Pulido L, Ghanem E, Joshi A, et al. Periprosthetic joint infection: the incidence, timing, and predisposing factors. Clin Orthop Relat Res 2008;466:1710–5.
23. Greenky M, Gandhi K, Pulido L, et al. Preoperative anemia in total joint arthroplasty: is it associated with periprosthetic joint infection? Clin Orthop Relat Res 2012;470:2695–701.

24. Hsieh PH, Huang KC, Shih HN. Prosthetic joint infection in patients with rheumatoid arthritis: an outcome analysis compared with controls. PLoS One 2013;8: e71666.
25. Carpenter MT, West SG, Vogelgesang SA, et al. Postoperative joint infections in rheumatoid arthritis patients on methotrexate therapy. Orthopedics 1996;19: 207–10.
26. Bongartz T. Elective orthopedic surgery and perioperative DMARD management: many questions, fewer answers, and some opinions. J Rheumatol 2007;34:653–5.
27. Grennan DM, Gray J, Loudon J, et al. Methotrexate and early postoperative complications in patients with rheumatoid arthritis undergoing elective orthopaedic surgery. Ann Rheum Dis 2001;60:214–7.
28. Ding T, Ledingham J, Luqmani R, et al. BSR and BHPR rheumatoid arthritis guidelines on safety of anti-TNF therapies. Rheumatology (Oxford) 2010;49:2217–9.
29. Marculescu CE, Mabry T, Berbari EF. Prevention of surgical site infections in joint replacement surgery. Surg Infect (Larchmt) 2016;17:152–7.
30. Tande AJ, Patel R. Prosthetic joint infection. Clin Microbiol Rev 2014;27:302–45.
31. Peel TN, Cheng AC, Buising KL, et al. Microbiological aetiology, epidemiology, and clinical profile of prosthetic joint infections: are current antibiotic prophylaxis guidelines effective? Antimicrob Agents Chemother 2012;56:2386–91.
32. Kourbatova EV, Halvosa JS, King MD, et al. Emergence of community-associated methicillin-resistant Staphylococcus aureus USA 300 clone as a cause of health care-associated infections among patients with prosthetic joint infections. Am J Infect Control 2005;33:385–91.
33. Kalmeijer MD, Coertjens H, van Nieuwland-Bollen PM, et al. Surgical site infections in orthopedic surgery: the effect of mupirocin nasal ointment in a double-blind, randomized, placebo-controlled study. Clin Infect Dis 2002;35:353–8.
34. Hacek DM, Robb WJ, Paule SM, et al. Staphylococcus aureus nasal decolonization in joint replacement surgery reduces infection. Clin Orthop Relat Res 2008; 466:1349–55.
35. Zywiel MG, Daley JA, Delanois RE, et al. Advance pre-operative chlorhexidine reduces the incidence of surgical site infections in knee arthroplasty. Int Orthop 2011;35:1001–6.
36. Johnson AJ, Daley JA, Zywiel MG, et al. Preoperative chlorhexidine preparation and the incidence of surgical site infections after hip arthroplasty. J Arthroplasty 2010;25:98–102.
37. Farber NJ, Chen AF, Bartsch SM, et al. No infection reduction using chlorhexidine wipes in total joint arthroplasty. Clin Orthop Relat Res 2013;471:3120–5.
38. Bode LG, Kluytmans JA, Wertheim HF, et al. Preventing surgical-site infections in nasal carriers of Staphylococcus aureus. N Engl J Med 2010;362:9–17.
39. Bratzler DW, Dellinger EP, Olsen KM, et al. Clinical practice guidelines for antimicrobial prophylaxis in surgery. Am J Health Syst Pharm 2013;70:195–283.
40. Baratz MD, Hallmark R, Odum SM, et al. Twenty percent of patients may remain colonized with methicillin-resistant Staphylococcus aureus despite a decolonization protocol in patients undergoing elective total joint arthroplasty. Clin Orthop Relat Res 2015;473:2283–90.
41. Economedes DM, Deirmengian GK, Deirmengian CA. Staphylococcus aureus colonization among arthroplasty patients previously treated by a decolonization protocol: a pilot study. Clin Orthop Relat Res 2013;471:3128–32.
42. Fogelberg EV, Zitzmann EK, Stinchfield FE. Prophylactic penicillin in orthopaedic surgery. J Bone Joint Surg Am 1970;52:95–8.

43. AlBuhairan B, Hind D, Hutchinson A. Antibiotic prophylaxis for wound infections in total joint arthroplasty: a systematic review. J Bone Joint Surg Br 2008;90:915–9.

44. Walsh EE, Greene L, Kirshner R. Sustained reduction in methicillin-resistant staphylococcus aureus wound infections after cardiothoracic surgery. Arch Intern Med 2011;171:68–73.

45. Garey KW, Lai D, Dao-Tran TK, et al. Interrupted time series analysis of vancomycin compared to cefuroxime for surgical prophylaxis in patients undergoing cardiac surgery. Antimicrob Agents Chemother 2008;52:446–51.

46. Finkelstein R, Rabino G, Mashiah T, et al. Vancomycin versus cefazolin prophylaxis for cardiac surgery in the setting of a high prevalence of methicillin-resistant staphylococcal infections. J Thorac Cardiovasc Surg 2002;123:326–32.

47. Sewick A, Makani A, Wu C, et al. Does dual antibiotic prophylaxis better prevent surgical site infections in total joint arthroplasty? Clin Orthop Relat Res 2012;470: 2702–7.

48. Ho VP, Nicolau DP, Dakin GF, et al. Cefazolin dosing for surgical prophylaxis in morbidly obese patients. Surg Infect (Larchmt) 2012;13:33–7.

49. Unger NR, Stein BJ. Effectiveness of pre-operative cefazolin in obese patients. Surg Infect (Larchmt) 2014;15:412–6.

50. Rybak MJ, Lomaestro BM, Rotschafer JC, et al. Vancomycin therapeutic guidelines: a summary of consensus recommendations from the Infectious Diseases Society of America, the American Society of Health-System Pharmacists, and the Society of Infectious Diseases Pharmacists. Clin Infect Dis 2009;49:325–7.

51. Nelson CL, Green TG, Porter RA, et al. One day versus seven days of preventive antibiotic therapy in orthopedic surgery. Clin Orthop Relat Res 1983;(176):258–63.

52. Parvizi J, Saleh KJ, Ragland PS, et al. Efficacy of antibiotic-impregnated cement in total hip replacement. Acta Orthop 2008;79:335–41.

53. Wang J, Zhu C, Cheng T, et al. A systematic review and meta-analysis of antibiotic-impregnated bone cement use in primary total hip or knee arthroplasty. PLoS One 2013;8:e82745.

54. van Kasteren ME, Mannien J, Ott A, et al. Antibiotic prophylaxis and the risk of surgical site infections following total hip arthroplasty: timely administration is the most important factor. Clin Infect Dis 2007;44:921–7.

55. Goodman SB, Yao Z, Keeney M, et al. The future of biologic coatings for orthopaedic implants. Biomaterials 2013;34:3174–83.

56. Dumville JC, McFarlane E, Edwards P, et al. Preoperative skin antiseptics for preventing surgical wound infections after clean surgery. Cochrane Database Syst Rev 2015;(4):CD003949.

57. Webster J, Alghamdi A. Use of plastic adhesive drapes during surgery for preventing surgical site infection. Cochrane Database Syst Rev 2015;(4):CD006353.

58. James M, Khan WS, Nannaparaju MR, et al. Current evidence for the use of laminar flow in reducing infection rates in total joint arthroplasty. Open Orthop J 2015;9:495–8.

59. Gastmeier P, Breier AC, Brandt C. Influence of laminar airflow on prosthetic joint infections: a systematic review. J Hosp Infect 2012;81:73–8.

60. Andersson AE, Bergh I, Karlsson J, et al. Traffic flow in the operating room: an explorative and descriptive study on air quality during orthopedic trauma implant surgery. Am J Infect Control 2012;40:750–5.

61. Bedard M, Pelletier-Roy R, Angers-Goulet M, et al. Traffic in the operating room during joint replacement is a multidisciplinary problem. Can J Surg 2015;58: 232–6.

62. Panahi P, Stroh M, Casper DS, et al. Operating room traffic is a major concern during total joint arthroplasty. Clin Orthop Relat Res 2012;470:2690–4.

63. Sousa R, Munoz-Mahamud E, Quayle J, et al. Is asymptomatic bacteriuria a risk factor for prosthetic joint infection? Clin Infect Dis 2014;59:41–7.

64. Berbari EF, Osmon DR, Carr A, et al. Dental procedures as risk factors for prosthetic hip or knee infection: a hospital-based prospective case-control study. Clin Infect Dis 2010;50:8–16.

65. Bartzokas CA, Johnson R, Jane M, et al. Relation between mouth and haematogenous infection in total joint replacements. BMJ 1994;309:506–8.

66. Gupta A, Osmon DR, Hanssen AD, et al. Genitourinary procedures as risk factors for prosthetic hip or knee infection: a hospital-based prospective case-control study. Open Forum Infect Dis 2015;2:ofv097.

67. Coelho-Prabhu N, Oxentenko AS, Osmon DR, et al. Increased risk of prosthetic joint infection associated with esophago-gastro-duodenoscopy with biopsy. Acta Orthop 2013;84:82–6.

68. Saleh K, Olson M, Resig S, et al. Predictors of wound infection in hip and knee joint replacement: results from a 20 year surveillance program. J Orthop Res 2002;20:506–15.

69. Galat DD, McGovern SC, Larson DR, et al. Surgical treatment of early wound complications following primary total knee arthroplasty. J Bone Joint Surg Am 2009;91:48–54.

70. Zingg M, Miozzari HH, Fritschy D, et al. Influence of body mass index on revision rates after primary total knee arthroplasty. Int Orthop 2016;40:723–9.

71. Kunutsor SK, Whitehouse MR, Blom AW, et al. Patient-related risk factors for periprosthetic joint infection after total joint arthroplasty: a systematic review and meta-analysis. PLoS One 2016;11:e0150866.

72. Jamsen E, Huhtala H, Puolakka T, et al. Risk factors for infection after knee arthroplasty. A register-based analysis of 43,149 cases. J Bone Joint Surg Am 2009;91:38–47.

73. Poss R, Thornhill TS, Ewald FC, et al. Factors influencing the incidence and outcome of infection following total joint arthroplasty. Clin Orthop Relat Res 1984;(182):117–26.

74. Espehaug B, Furnes O, Havelin LI, et al. The type of cement and failure of total hip replacements. J Bone Joint Surg Br 2002;84:832–8.

75. Racano A, Pazionis T, Farrokhyar F, et al. High infection rate outcomes in long-bone tumor surgery with endoprosthetic reconstruction in adults: a systematic review. Clin Orthop Relat Res 2013;471:2017–27.

76. Dalstrom DJ, Venkatarayappa I, Manternach AL, et al. Time-dependent contamination of opened sterile operating-room trays. J Bone Joint Surg Am 2008;90:1022–5.

77. Hadley S, Immerman I, Hutzler L, et al. Staphylococcus aureus decolonization protocol decreases surgical site infections for total joint replacement. Arthritis 2010;2010:924518.

78. Melling AC, Ali B, Scott EM, et al. Effects of preoperative warming on the incidence of wound infection after clean surgery: a randomised controlled trial. Lancet 2001;358:876–80.

79. Putzu M, Casati A, Berti M, et al. Clinical complications, monitoring and management of perioperative mild hypothermia: anesthesiological features. Acta Biomed 2007;78:163–9.

80. Tanner J, Norrie P, Melen K. Preoperative hair removal to reduce surgical site infection. Cochrane Database Syst Rev 2011;(11):CD004122.

81. Zhou X, Yishake M, Li J, et al. Genetic susceptibility to prosthetic joint infection following total joint arthroplasty: a systematic review. Gene 2015;563:76–82.
82. Darouiche RO, Wall MJ Jr, Itani KM, et al. Chlorhexidine-alcohol versus povidone-iodine for surgical-site antisepsis. N Engl J Med 2010;362:18–26.
83. Markatos K, Kaseta M, Nikolaou VS. Perioperative skin preparation and draping in modern total joint arthroplasty: current evidence. Surg Infect (Larchmt) 2015; 16:221–5.

Reactive Arthritis

Steven K. Schmitt, MD

KEYWORDS

- Reactive arthritis • Inflammatory arthritis • Spondyloarthropathy • Chlamydia
- Salmonella • Shigella • Yersinia • Campylobacter

KEY POINTS

- Reactive arthritis is categorized as a spondyloarthropathy. Pathogenesis involves a gastrointestinal or genitourinary infectious trigger in the susceptible host.
- Clinical presentation is of a monoarthritis or oligoarthritis, usually of the lower extremities. Other musculoskeletal manifestations include enthesitis and dactylitis.
- Antibiotic therapy provides benefit in the setting of chlamydial infection; the role of antibiotics for enteric pathogens is less clear.
- Anti-inflammatory treatment is initiated with nonsteroidal antiinflammatory drugs. Refractory disease is treated with nonbiological disease-modifying agents. The role of tumor necrosis factor alpha inhibitors is evolving.
- Many patients experience a clinical course measured in a few months, but some go on to more severe and chronic courses.

INTRODUCTION

Reactive arthritis is typically defined as an inflammatory arthritis not directly caused by culture-proven infection of joint tissue, but rather after infection at another site. Historically, the term "Reiter's syndrome" was often used as synonymous. Over time, it has become recognized that Reiter's syndrome is a subset of reactive arthritis. In addition, there is some controversy surrounding the use of the term Reiter's syndrome, in light of the role of its namesake in Nazi medical experimentation.[1] The disease is now commonly included in the category of spondyloarthropathies, accounting for less than 2% of the overall disease burden in this category in 1 study.[2] Patients often present to primary care physicians, and multidisciplinary care including rheumatology and infectious diseases specialists is frequently required.

Clinical Criteria

There are no agreed upon, validated diagnostic criteria for reactive arthritis.[3] Proposed definitions[4] have included a combination of microbiological and clinical criteria (**Box 1**). Reiter's syndrome was classically defined as the triad of arthritis, urethritis,

The author has no relevant disclosures.
Section of Bone and Joint Infections, Department of Infectious Disease, Medicine Institute, Cleveland Clinic Lerner College of Medicine, Cleveland Clinic, 9500 Euclid Avenue, Desk G-21, Cleveland, OH 44195, USA
E-mail address: schmits@ccf.org

Infect Dis Clin N Am 31 (2017) 265–277
http://dx.doi.org/10.1016/j.idc.2017.01.002
0891-5520/17/© 2017 Elsevier Inc. All rights reserved.

id.theclinics.com

> **Box 1**
> **Criteria for reactive arthritis**
>
> 1. Arthritis after microbiologically confirmed enteric or genitourinary infection after a period of days to weeks, with clinical or laboratory evidence of infection.
> 2. Asymmetric monoarthritis or oligoarthritis usually of the lower extremities.
> 3. No other cause for arthritis such as septic arthritis or crystalline arthropathy.

and conjunctivitis. In 1 study, an episode of arthritis of more than 1 month's duration, combined with urethritis and/or cervicitis, had an 84% sensitivity and 98% specificity for this syndrome.[5]

Acute reactive arthritis typically lasts 6 months or less in one-half of patients and symptoms resolve for most in 1 year. Patients with symptoms that exceed this duration are said to have chronic reactive arthritis.

MICROBIOLOGY

Reactive arthritis typically arises after an infection with gastrointestinal or genitourinary bacterial pathogens (**Box 2**).

Chlamydia trachomatis is strongly associated with reactive arthritis. Nucleic acid from this organism has been detected in synovial fluid by direct immunofluorescence or polymerase chain reaction.[6] Gastrointestinal pathogens such as *Campylobacter jejuni, Clostridium difficile, Escherichia coli, Salmonella* (various species), *Shigella* (especially *S flexneri*), *and Yersinia* (especially *Y enterocolitica* and *Y pseudotuberculosis*). Respiratory pathogens such as *Chlamydia pneumoniae*[7] or *Mycoplasma pneumoniae*[8] have also been shown to give rise to reactive joint processes. Reactive arthritis may occur in the setting of human immunodeficiency virus infection, although human immunodeficiency virus is usually not directly associated and other pathogens are usually implicated.[9]

EPIDEMIOLOGY

Reactive arthritis typically occurs in sporadic cases, but may occur with increased frequency in the setting of outbreaks of infection. A systematic review of incidence of

> **Box 2**
> **Inciting agents of reactive arthritis**
>
> *Common*
>
> *Chlamydia trachomatis*
>
> *Salmonella* (several species)
>
> *Shigella* (especially *S flexneri*)
>
> *Campylobacter jejuni*
>
> *Yersinia* (especially *Y enterocolitica* and *Y pseudotuberculosis*)
>
> *Uncommon*
>
> *Chlamydophila pneumoniae*
>
> Human immunodeficiency virus
>
> *Clostridium difficile*

reactive arthritis with enteric pathogens[10] revealed 9 cases per 1000 *Campylobacter* infections, 12 cases per 1000 *Salmonella* infections, and 12 cases per 1000 *Shigella* infections. Reactive arthritis complicates 1.4% of cases of *C difficile* infection in children.[11] Epidemiologic data on the incidence of reactive arthritis after genital chlamydia infection suggests an incidence of 4% to 8%. Relative risk for development of reactive arthritis is higher among women (relative risk 1.5 vs males) and adults (relative risk 2.5 vs children) for the enteric form of the disease.[12]

PATHOGENESIS

As it is currently understood, reactive arthritis is a complex interplay of host antimicrobial factors. There has been considerable focus on the role of HLA-B27 in reactive arthritis, which has yet to be completely clarified. HLA-B27 is positive in 50% to 80% of patients with reactive arthritis.[13] HLA-B27–carrying individuals are felt to have a higher incidence of reactive arthritis, although the predominance of HLA-B27 in populations with reactive arthritis varies somewhat. In 1 study, HLA-B27 positive patients had more a severe acute disease course with a longer duration of symptoms, more extraarticular symptoms, and more chronic symptoms.[14] HLA-B27 has also been strongly associated with pathogenesis of spondyloarthropathy; with inflammation at the entheses, where ligaments, tendons, cartilage, and joint capsules meet; and with bony ankylosis of the sacroiliac and spinal facet joints. HLA-B2705 is the subtype most commonly associated with spondyloarthropathies.

Several hypotheses have evolved to explain the role of HLA-B27 in these processes. The HLA-B27 misfolding hypothesis[15] observes that HLA-B27 folds more slowly than other HLA types as it is assembled in the endoplasmic reticulum. This slow pace is felt to lead to improper folding and instability of HLA-B27, with accumulation of HLA-B27 homodimers and beta-2 microglobulin, with activation of inflammatory processes.

The arthritogenic peptide hypothesis[16] relies on aberrant antigen presentation in pathogenesis. It states that microbial peptides mimic certain self-peptides, causing reactivity of HLA-B27 specific, CD8 bearing cytotoxic T lymphocytes. It is suggested that this then leads to autoimmunity and inflammation with tissue damage.

The heavy chain homodimer hypothesis[17] observes that HLA-B27 may be expressed on the cell surface as homodimers of heavy chains without beta-2 microglobulin. These heavy chains then activate natural killer cells, T cells, and B cells, with inflammatory consequences for the surrounding tissue.

Because some patients who are HLA-B27 negative also develop reactive arthritis, other investigations have focused on the role of microbial factors in pathogenesis. One recent study of patients with reactive arthritis due to *S typhimurium* suggests that *Salmonella* outer membrane protein is able to stimulate interleukin (IL)-17/IL-23 production in synovial immune cells, possibly contributing to arthropathy.[18]

There is evolving evidence that some forms of reactive arthritis may be related to persistence of the underlying infection in some subsets of the disease. Gerard and colleagues[19] were able to demonstrate the presence of metabolically active (having active messenger RNA secretion) *C trachomatis* in the synovial tissue of 4 patients with chronic reactive arthritis attributable to the organism. There is also evidence that differences in expression of heat shock protein-60 genes may contribute to organism persistence.[20]

Additional studies have focused on the role of the gastrointestinal microbiota in the pathogenesis of spondyloarthropathies. One proposed model suggests that the altered microbiota can in turn lead to aberrant immune responses to gut flora, loss of gut homeostasis, inflammation, and subsequently to spondyloarthropathy.[21]

CLINICAL PRESENTATION
Primary Infection

Genitourinary infection with *C trachomatis* typically presents as cervicitis in women, but may also present as pelvic inflammatory disease.[22] The most common presentation in men is urethritis, but epididymitis is also observed.[23] The discharge caused by *Chlamydia* is usually mucopurulent but may be clear, and is often present in small amounts.

Gastrointestinal infection with *S enteritidis* or *S typhimurium* presents with diarrhea and fever, although both may be relatively mild. *Salmonella* can infect bones and joints, so it is important to exclude septic arthritis or osteomyelitis with these organisms. Leukopenia may be present in the initial infection. In reactive arthritis, joint symptoms follow acute enteric infection by 1 to 3 weeks.

Enteric infections with *Shigella* species tend to be more acute, with bloody diarrhea accompanied by high-grade fever.[24] Arthritis may be delayed by a few weeks to several months. *Yersinia* infections presented with a fever, diarrhea, and right lower quadrant tenderness.[25] The acute gastroenteritis may be followed within 1 to 2 weeks by arthritis. *Campylobacter* causes a moderate diarrhea and may develop reactive arthritis in 10 to 14 days.[10]

Musculoskeletal Manifestations

Reactive arthritis presents as a peripheral monoarthritis or asymmetric oligoarthritis, enthesitis or dactylitis (**Box 3**).[3,26] The onset of symptoms is days to several weeks after the inciting infection. Symptoms of the inciting infection have often resolved by the time of onset of musculoskeletal signs and symptoms.

Reactive arthritis typically occurs in the lower extremities, although upper extremity involvement, including the small joints of the hands, is not uncommon.[27] Involvement of the axial skeleton is less common, affecting sacroiliac joints, the lumbar spine, or less commonly the thoracic or cervical spine. Joint manifestations may be sequential rather than simultaneous. Low back pain is a common accompanying symptom. Mild warmth and large joint effusion may be present.

Enthesitis is inflammation at the enthesis, which is the insertion point to bone of the tendons, ligaments, fascia, or capsule. Lower extremity involvement with Achilles tendinitis or plantar fasciitis is the usual presentation, but knee and upper extremity sites may be seen.[27] This feature is common in reactive arthritis and helps to distinguish from other differential diagnoses.

Box 3
Musculoskeletal manifestations of reactive arthritis

Peripheral

Monoarthritis or asymmetric > symmetric oligoarthritis (especially large joints of lower extremities)

Enthesitis (tendon/bone insertion points—Achilles tendonitis or plantar fasciitis > knees or upper extremities)

Dactylitis (sausage digit fingers or toes)

Axial

Spine (lumbar > thoracic/cervical)

Sacroiliac joints

Dactylitis, also known as sausage digit, is painful inflammation of an entire finger or toe. Dactylitis occurs in up to 40% of some populations with reactive arthritis,[27] and is a common feature for spondyloarthropathies.

Extraarticular Manifestations

Extraarticular manifestations are not rare, particularly in the setting of genitourinary infection (**Box 4**).[28] Genitourinary symptoms may include urethritis (part of the traditional syndrome), cervicitis, salpingo-oophoritis, cystitis (with sterile urine), or prostatitis.[29] Symptoms may be secondary to the underlying infection, especially with *Chlamydia*.

Ophthalmologic symptoms include conjunctivitis (again, part of the traditional triad), keratitis, episcleritis, or anterior uveitis.[28] Mucocutaneous manifestations include oral ulceration, and skin eruptions such as erythema nodosum and keratoderma blennorrhagica. Genital lesions include circinate balanitis. Skin lesions tend to occur with prolonged disease. In 1 review,[30] all of the case patients had joint systems for at least 1 month and most several months to years before the development of skin lesions.

Cardiac manifestations have been reported and may include aortic valvular insufficiency, heart block,[31,32] and pericarditis.[33] Pericarditis tends to occur with longer duration of illness, and valvular disease and heart block may occur early in the course.

DIAGNOSIS

The most convincing diagnosis of reactive arthritis relies on the detection of the appropriate trigger in the genetically susceptible host with a compatible clinical syndrome (**Box 5**).

History and Physical Examination

A careful history will elicit symptomatology of prior infection, often diarrhea or dysuria, as well as musculoskeletal pain. Physical examination can yield evidence of musculoskeletal infection, with joint effusions and tenderness, tender entheses, and dactylitis. Examination findings indicative of extraarticular disease may include genitourinary signs such as urethral discharge or circinate balanitis. Mucocutaneous signs such as keratoderma blennorrhagica or oral ulceration may be present. Injection or pain may herald inflammatory eye involvement as described. Acute onset of heart murmur or rub is rarely found, but may indicate significant cardiac complications.

Confirmation of Triggering Infection

A cornerstone of diagnosis is a good faith attempt to confirm the triggering infection, although sensitivity of testing is often 50% or less.[34,35] A combination of enzyme immunoassay and culture of stool is usually used to detect enteric pathogens, such

---

Box 4
Extraarticular manifestations of reactive arthritis

Genitourinary: Urethritis, cervicitis, salpingo-oophoritis, cystitis, prostatitis

Mucous membranes: Painless oral ulceration

Cutaneous: Keratoderma blennorrhagica, circinate balanitis, erythema nodosum

Ophthalmologic: Conjunctivitis, keratitis, episcleritis, or anterior uveitis

Cardiac: Aortic valvular insufficiency, pericarditis, heart block

> **Box 5**
> **Diagnosis of reactive arthritis**
>
> History and physical examination
>   Prior infection, articular and extraarticular manifestations
>
> Confirmation of triggering infection
>   *Enteric:* Stool culture/enzyme immunoassay: *Campylobacter, Salmonella, Shigella,* or *Yersinia*
>   *Polymerase chain reaction:* C difficile
>   *Genitourinary:* nucleic acid amplification of urine or a urethral swab—*Chlamydia trachomatis*
>
> HLA–B27 testing
>
> Acute phase reactants
>   Modest with genitourinary source; higher when enthesitis present
>
> Synovial fluid analysis
>   5000 to 50,000 white blood cells per high-powered field; predominance of neutrophils, negative cultures
>
> Imaging
>   *Plain radiographs:* soft tissue swelling, irregular periosteum at entheses; osteopenia, bony spur formation or joint erosion in chronic disease
>   *MRI:* sacroiliac bone edema and inflammation, contrast enhancement of synovia or entheses

as *Campylobacter, Salmonella, Shigella,* or *Yersinia*. Stool polymerase chain reaction is the most frequent tool used to diagnose *C difficile* infection. In a like fashion, nucleic acid amplification of urine or a urethral swab specimen is most commonly used to diagnose *C trachomatis* infection. Antibody testing may also be used to identify in particular, but positive serologies often do not distinguish between remote and recent infection. In addition, serology results are often delayed by several days after collection, limiting clinical usefulness.

Testing for HLA-B27

HLA-B27 is found in 50% to 80% of patients with reactive arthritis. A positive blood test supports the diagnosis in the appropriate clinical setting.

Acute Phase Reactants

The erythrocyte sedimentation rate and C-reactive protein are often, but not invariably, elevated. These usually correlate with the platelet count, which is elevated. Acute phase reactants tends to be higher when enthesitis is present in spondyloarthropathy.[35] Patients with chlamydial reactive arthritis tend to have lower acute phase reactant values compared with those with nonchlamydial reactive arthritis.[36] Patients with long-standing arthritis may have anemia in a chronic disease pattern.

Synovial Fluid Analysis

Synovial fluid is usually suggestive of an inflammatory arthritis with pleocytosis generally in the range of 10,000 to 50,000 WBC per high-powered field and with a predominance of neutrophils. In this range, there is considerable overlap with many other inflammatory conditions.[37] Given that infection is in the differential diagnosis, it is reasonable to send fluid for Gram stain and culture. Molecular amplification is usually not necessary.

Imaging Findings

Radiographic findings seen in reactive arthritis tend to be nonspecific. Plain radiographs may show soft tissue swelling or irregular periosteum at sites of entheses, such as the Achilles tendon and plantar fascia. Ultrasound examination of the Achilles tendon shows bursal thickening in spondyloarthritis.[38] MRI findings in spondyloarthropathy may include sacroiliac bone edema and inflammation, and contrast enhancement characteristic of synovitis or enthesitis in symptomatic patients.[39] More long-standing disease may reveal osteopenia, bony spur formation, or joint erosion.

DIFFERENTIAL DIAGNOSIS

The differential diagnosis of acute monoarthritis or oligoarthritis is broad (**Box 6**). Septic arthritis (described in John J. Ross's article, "Septic Arthritis of Native Joints," in this issue) is critical to exclude, given the morbidity of the disease with joint destruction and need for urgent washout and antibiotic therapy. Considering mimics of the reactive arthritis clinical syndrome, disseminated gonococcal infection is a treatable disease with genitourinary symptoms followed by inflammatory arthritis and pustular or maculopapular rash.[40] Like reactive arthritis, patients with disseminated gonococcal infection can also have heel pain, in this case caused by Achilles tenosynovitis. In these entities, fever and leukocytosis are common, whereas it is less common in reactive arthritis. Nucleic acid amplification of genitourinary samples is used commonly for diagnosis. Synovial fluid examination with routine analysis, Gram stain, and culture are essential to the evaluation of septic arthritis and gonococcal infection.

Enteroviral infections such as those caused by Coxsackie virus[41,42] and echovirus commonly cause diarrhea and may cause inflammatory arthritis in a small minority of cases. Constitutional symptoms of viral infection including fever and myalgia can help differentiate from reactive arthritis.

Whipple's disease, a treatable bacterial infection caused by *Tropheryma whippeli*, causes diarrhea, and may be accompanied by an acute oligoarthritis or chronic polyarthritis.[43] The presence of central nervous system disease or endocarditis, which can complicate Whipple's disease, can help to differentiate it from reactive arthropathy.

When arthritis complicates a longer standing diarrhea, inflammatory bowel diseases such as Crohn's disease and ulcerative colitis should be considered. Behçets disease may be complicated by diarrhea and arthritis, along with the more common skin and

---

Box 6
Differential diagnosis of reactive arthritis

Septic arthritis (inflammatory monoarthritis or oligoarthritis)

Disseminated gonococcal infection (genitourinary symptoms, arthritis)

Enteroviral infection (diarrhea, arthritis)

Whipple's disease (acute oligoarthritis or chronic polyarthritis)

Inflammatory bowel disease (diarrhea, arthritis)

Behçets disease (diarrhea, arthritis, skin and genital ulcers, rash, uveitis)

Crystalline arthropathy

Lyme disease

Poststreptococcal arthritis

genital ulcers, rash, and uveitis. Joint pain can accompany the significant, malabsorption-related diarrhea of celiac disease.

Other noninfectious differential diagnoses include crystalline arthropathies with urate (gout) or calcium pyrophosphate (pseudogout). In the correct epidemiologic setting, testing for Lyme disease, which can cause rash and arthritis, can yield another important alternative diagnosis treated with antimicrobial therapy. Postinfectious arthritis may complicate group A streptococcal disease. These manifestations occur in a spectrum that ranges from the migratory polyarthritis that is part of Jones' criteria for acute rheumatic fever, to the more limited post-streptococcal arthritis.[44] Detection of group A streptococci by throat swab for culture or molecular testing, or streptococcal antibody testing, supports these diagnoses.

MANAGEMENT

The appropriate management of reactive arthritis must consider treatment of the underlying infection and articular and extraarticular disease manifestations. The evidence for treatment of the underlying infection varies by the type of infection. To date, there is no convincing evidence that treatment of gastrointestinal infection alters the course of reactive arthritis. A metaanalysis of available studies showed no improvement in remission of symptoms, and antibiotic therapy led to double the rate of gastrointestinal side effects of treatment.[45] Also, antibiotics are not generally recommended for mild to moderate bacterial enteric infection, with or without reactive arthropathy. However, antibiotic therapy may be warranted for severe bacterial gastrointestinal infection in patients relatively immune compromised by age, disease, or immunosuppressive treatment.

Conversely, patients with reactive arthritis triggered by C trachomatis may benefit from a course of antibiotic therapy. Although the duration of treatment is a source of discussion, 6 months of oral antibiotic therapy with either doxycycline or azithromycin, both combined with rifampin, has been shown to improve joint symptoms for 63% patients compared with 20% with placebo, and to remission in 22% receiving antibiotics, compared with none of patients receiving placebo.[46]

Data on the treatment of the articular symptoms of reactive arthritis are lacking. In general, goals of therapy are to reduce pain, swelling, and tenderness. Initial treatment of acute reactive arthritis is usually with antiinflammatory doses of nonsteroidal antiinflammatory drugs (NSAIDs),[26] for a minimum of 2 weeks before assessing response. Naproxen 500 mg twice a day has a good side effects profile in short-term use. A 2-week course may be sufficient, given the self-limited natural history of acute reactive arthritis in many patients. Treatment doses of NSAIDs have a potential for side effects, which should be included in patient education in this setting. Indeed, boxed warnings are included in drug instructions in the United States regarding the potential for cardiovascular thrombotic events and gastrointestinal bleeding. Prolonged high-dose NSAID therapy can also lead to kidney and hepatic injury, in addition to cardiac events. Risks and benefits should be especially considered and discussed with patients who have preexisting renal, hepatic, and cardiac disease. Regular laboratory monitoring should be part of treatment and include hepatic and renal function, as well as a complete blood count.

Inadequate response of articular symptoms to or intolerance of NSAIDs in patients with acute reactive arthritis should lead to consideration for intraarticular glucocorticoid therapy. Intraarticular glucocorticoids, such as triamcinolone, provide symptomatic relief and spare potential side effects of systemic steroids.

Systemic glucocorticoids are used when the patient does not respond to NSAIDs or intraarticular glucocorticoids or has a large number of involved joints. With no clear-cut data on dose or duration available, practitioners often rely on the severity of arthritis to guide choice of dose, in the range of prednisone 20 mg/d for mild disease and 40 mg/d or higher for moderate to severe disease. The dose should be tapered appropriately to the lowest effective dose, given the significant adverse effects profile with prolonged use of higher doses, including susceptibility to infection and osteopenia. Nonbiological disease-modifying antirheumatic drugs (DMARDs) may be used for acute reactive arthritis unresponsive to NSAIDs or glucocorticoid therapy.

Chronic Reactive Arthritis

Because NSAIDs and glucocorticoids are most often used for several weeks to months before considering an escalation in therapy, DMARDs are typically used in chronic forms of the disease. The 2 DMARDs most commonly used in this setting are sulfasalazine (SSZ) and methotrexate. SSZ is the better studied of the 2 agents. Its efficacy is of pathogenetic interest because of the gastrointestinal disease trigger and finding of bowel inflammation in a significant percentage of patients with reactive arthritis. In 1 placebo-controlled, prospective study, there was a strong trend without statistical significance toward response (as defined by improvement in patient inclination assessment of joint pain, tenderness, and swelling) in patients treated with SSZ (62%) over those treated with placebo (47%).[47] Dosing in this study for treated patients consisted of 500 mg of SSZ for 1 week, increased by 500 mg/d each week until a total of 2000 mg/d was reached. Adverse events are relatively common. Treatment limiting events may include gastrointestinal upset, central nervous system toxicity, and rash. A syndrome of rash, fever, and abnormal hepatic transaminases occurs in fewer than 1% of treated patients, but may be serious and the drug should be immediately and permanently discontinued if recognized. Leukopenia and neutropenia may also occur and are often addressed by dose adjustment; agranulocytosis is another cause for immediate and permanent discontinuation. Glucose-6-phosphate dehydrogenase deficiency may lead to hemolytic anemia with use of SSZ and should be screened for before initiation of therapy. Laboratory monitoring should include a complete blood count with differential, hepatic transaminases, and creatinine every 2 to 4 weeks for the first 3 months of therapy, with frequency decreasing thereafter.

Methotrexate has been used as an alternative to SSZ when patients are unresponsive to or intolerant of NSAIDs, glucocorticoids, and SSZ. Although there are no study data supporting use in reactive arthritis, it has been used in ankylosing spondylitis with peripheral joint involvement.

It must be noted that nonbiological DMARDs are considered less effective in enthesitis or dactylitis.[48] If NSAIDs fail in these patients with these manifestations, consideration should be given to tumor necrosis factor inhibitor therapy.

Response to nonbiological DMARDs is determined by observation over a 3- to 4-month course of maximal doses of the drugs. Patients who respond continue therapy for 3 to 6 months after resolution of disease signs and symptoms and then are considered for discontinuation. Patients who fail to respond are considered for therapy with biological disease-modifying agents, typically the anti–tumor necrosis factor agents such as etanercept, adalimumab, or infliximab.[49–51] Data supporting the role of anti–tumor necrosis factor agents in reactive arthritis are limited to case reports and small series, with response in terms of symptoms or biochemical markers. In these series, patients were able to discontinue steroid therapy. Further studies are needed to confirm efficacy and assess potential concerns regarding exacerbation of the triggering infection.

Nonarticular manifestations of reactive arthritis may also require specific therapy. Because no treatment studies for reactive arthritis have addressed them specifically, expert consultative assistance with an ophthalmologist or dermatologist is essential. Oral ulceration may respond to topical steroid therapy. Skin manifestations such as keratoderma blennorrhagica and circinate balanitis may also respond to topical steroids. Anterior uveitis is typically treated with topical steroids, whereas posterior uveitis may require injected steroid solutions. Nonresponding disease is typically treated with systemic glucocorticoids or, in more refractory or severe symptomatology, biological or nonbiological DMARDs.

PROGNOSIS

The natural history of reactive arthritis suggests that most patients have complete or near complete remission within 6 to 12 months. By some estimates, 25% to 50% flare and require retreatment. Approximately 25% develop chronic disease and require ongoing or treatment.[52] Some of these patients develop signs and symptoms of ankylosing spondylitis, or inflammatory bowel disease.

REFERENCES

1. Panush RS, Wallace DJ, Dorff RE, et al. Retraction of the suggestion to use the term "Reiter's syndrome" sixty-five years later: the legacy of Reiter, a war criminal, should not be eponymic honor but rather condemnation. Arthritis Rheum 2007; 56(2):693-4.
2. Casals-Sanchez JL, Garcia De Yebenes Prous MJ, Descalzo Gallego MA, et al. Characteristics of patients with spondyloarthritis followed in rheumatology units in Spain. emAR II study. Reumatol Clin 2012;8(3):107-13.
3. Braun J, Kingsley G, van der Heijde D, et al. On the difficulties of establishing a consensus on the definition of and diagnostic investigations for reactive arthritis. Results and discussion of a questionnaire prepared for the 4th International Workshop on Reactive Arthritis, Berlin, Germany, July 3-6, 1999. J Rheumatol 2000;27(9):2185-92.
4. Kingsley G, Sieper J. Third International Workshop on Reactive Arthritis. 23-26 September 1995, Berlin, Germany. Report and abstracts. Ann Rheum Dis 1996;55(8):564-84.
5. Willkens RF, Arnett FC, Bitter T, et al. Reiter's syndrome. Evaluation of preliminary criteria for definite disease. Arthritis Rheum 1981;24(6):844-9.
6. Taylor-Robinson D, Gilroy CB, Thomas BJ, et al. Detection of Chlamydia trachomatis DNA in joints of reactive arthritis patients by polymerase chain reaction. Lancet 1992;340(8811):81-2.
7. Carter JD, Hudson AP. Recent advances and future directions in understanding and treating chlamydia-induced reactive arthritis. Expert Rev Clin Immunol 2017; 13(3):197-206.
8. Natarajan UR, Tan TL, Lau R. Reiter's disease following Mycoplasma pneumoniae infection. Int J STD AIDS 2001;12(5):349-50.
9. Adizie T, Moots RJ, Hodkinson B, et al. Inflammatory arthritis in HIV positive patients: a practical guide. BMC Infect Dis 2016;16:100.
10. Ajene AN, Fischer Walker CL, Black RE. Enteric pathogens and reactive arthritis: a systematic review of Campylobacter, Salmonella and Shigella-associated reactive arthritis. J Health Popul Nutr 2013;31(3):299-307.

11. Horton DB, Strom BL, Putt ME, et al. Epidemiology of Clostridium difficile infection-associated reactive arthritis in children: an underdiagnosed, potentially morbid condition. JAMA Pediatr 2016;170(7):e160217.
12. Townes JM, Deodhar AA, Laine ES, et al. Reactive arthritis following culture-confirmed infections with bacterial enteric pathogens in Minnesota and Oregon: a population-based study. Ann Rheum Dis 2008;67(12):1689–96.
13. Sieper J. Pathogenesis of reactive arthritis. Curr Rheumatol Rep 2001;3(5):412–8.
14. Leirisalo M, Skylv G, Kousa M, et al. Followup study on patients with Reiter's disease and reactive arthritis, with special reference to HLA-B27. Arthritis Rheum 1982;25(3):249–59.
15. Colbert RA, Tran TM, Layh-Schmitt G. HLA-B27 misfolding and ankylosing spondylitis. Mol Immunol 2014;57(1):44–51.
16. Sieper J. Disease mechanisms in reactive arthritis. Curr Rheumatol Rep 2004; 6(2):110–6.
17. Allen RL, O'Callaghan CA, McMichael AJ, et al. Cutting edge: HLA-B27 can form a novel beta 2-microglobulin-free heavy chain homodimer structure. J Immunol 1999;162(9):5045–8.
18. Chaurasia S, Shasany AK, Aggarwal A, et al. Recombinant salmonella typhimurium outer membrane protein A is recognized by synovial fluid CD8 cells and stimulates synovial fluid mononuclear cells to produce interleukin (IL)-17/IL-23 in patients with reactive arthritis and undifferentiated spondyloarthropathy. Clin Exp Immunol 2016;185(2):210–8.
19. Gerard HC, Carter JD, Hudson AP. Chlamydia trachomatis is present and metabolically active during the remitting phase in synovial tissues from patients with chronic chlamydia-induced reactive arthritis. Am J Med Sci 2013;346(1):22–5.
20. Carter JD, Inman RD, Whittum-Hudson J, et al. Chlamydia and chronic arthritis. Ann Med 2012;44(8):784–92.
21. Asquith M, Rosenbaum JT. The interaction between host genetics and the microbiome in the pathogenesis of spondyloarthropathies. Curr Opin Rheumatol 2016; 28(4):405–12.
22. Marrazzo JM. Mucopurulent cervicitis: no longer ignored, but still misunderstood. Infect Dis Clin North Am 2005;19(2):333–49, viii.
23. Moi H, Blee K, Horner PJ. Management of non-gonococcal urethritis. BMC Infect Dis 2015;15:294.
24. Porter CK, Choi D, Riddle MS. Pathogen-specific risk of reactive arthritis from bacterial causes of foodborne illness. J Rheumatol 2013;40(5):712–4.
25. Huovinen E, Sihvonen LM, Virtanen MJ, et al. Symptoms and sources of Yersinia enterocolitica-infection: a case-control study. BMC Infect Dis 2010;10:122.
26. Carter JD, Hudson AP. Reactive arthritis: clinical aspects and medical management. Rheum Dis Clin North Am 2009;35(1):21–44.
27. Collantes E, Zarco P, Munoz E, et al. Disease pattern of spondyloarthropathies in Spain: description of the first national registry (REGISPONSER) extended report. Rheumatology (Oxford) 2007;46(8):1309–15.
28. Kiss S, Letko E, Qamruddin S, et al. Long-term progression, prognosis, and treatment of patients with recurrent ocular manifestations of Reiter's syndrome. Ophthalmology 2003;110(9):1764–9.
29. Vilppula AH, Granfors KM, Yli-Kerttula UI. Infectious involvements in males with Reiter's syndrome. Clin Rheumatol 1984;3(4):443–9.
30. Kanwar AJ, Mahajan R. Reactive arthritis in India: a dermatologists' perspective. J Cutan Med Surg 2013;17(3):180–8.

31. Brown LE, Forfia P, Flynn JA. Aortic insufficiency in a patient with reactive arthritis: case report and review of the literature. HSS J 2011;7(2):187–9.

32. Cosh JA, Gerber N, Barritt DW, et al. Proceedings: cardiac lesions in Reiter's syndrome and ankylosing spondylitis. Ann Rheum Dis 1975;34(2):195.

33. Kanakoudi-Tsakalidou F, Pardalos G, Pratsidou-Gertsi P, et al. Persistent or severe course of reactive arthritis following Salmonella enteritidis infection. A prospective study of 9 cases. Scand J Rheumatol 1998;27(6):431–4.

34. Fendler C, Laitko S, Sorensen H, et al. Frequency of triggering bacteria in patients with reactive arthritis and undifferentiated oligoarthritis and the relative importance of the tests used for diagnosis. Ann Rheum Dis 2001;60(4): 337–43.

35. Carneiro S, Bortoluzzo A, Goncalves C, et al. Effect of enthesitis on 1505 Brazilian patients with spondyloarthritis. J Rheumatol 2013;40(10):1719–25.

36. Ozgul A, Dede I, Taskaynatan MA, et al. Clinical presentations of chlamydial and non-chlamydial reactive arthritis. Rheumatol Int 2006;26(10):879–85.

37. McCutchan HJ, Fisher RC. Synovial leukocytosis in infectious arthritis. Clin Orthop Relat Res 1990;257:226–30.

38. Falcao S, de Miguel E, Castillo-Gallego C, et al. Achilles enthesis ultrasound: the importance of the bursa in spondyloarthritis. Clin Exp Rheumatol 2013;31(3): 422–7.

39. Marzo-Ortega H, McGonagle D, O'Connor P, et al. Baseline and 1-year magnetic resonance imaging of the sacroiliac joint and lumbar spine in very early inflammatory back pain. relationship between symptoms, HLA-B27 and disease extent and persistence. Ann Rheum Dis 2009;68(11):1721–7.

40. Rice PA. Gonococcal arthritis (disseminated gonococcal infection). Infect Dis Clin North Am 2005;19(4):853–61.

41. Stewart CL, Chu EY, Introcaso CE, et al. Coxsackievirus A6-induced hand-foot-mouth disease. JAMA Dermatol 2013;149(12):1419–21.

42. Bhambhani V, Abraham J, Sahni M, et al. Outbreak of coxsackie B4 arthritis among newborns and staff of a neonatal unit. Trop Doct 2007;37(3):188–9.

43. Puechal X. Whipple's arthritis. Joint Bone Spine 2016;83(6):631–5.

44. van der Helm-van Mil AH. Acute rheumatic fever and poststreptococcal reactive arthritis reconsidered. Curr Opin Rheumatol 2010;22(4):437–42.

45. Barber CE, Kim J, Inman RD, et al. Antibiotics for treatment of reactive arthritis: a systematic review and metaanalysis. J Rheumatol 2013;40(6):916–28.

46. Carter JD, Espinoza LR, Inman RD, et al. Combination antibiotics as a treatment for chronic chlamydia-induced reactive arthritis: a double-blind, placebo-controlled, prospective trial. Arthritis Rheum 2010;62(5):1298–307.

47. Clegg DO, Reda DJ, Weisman MH, et al. Comparison of sulfasalazine and placebo in the treatment of reactive arthritis (Reiter's syndrome). A Department of Veterans Affairs cooperative study. Arthritis Rheum 1996;39(12):2021–7.

48. Sieper J, Poddubnyy D. New evidence on the management of spondyloarthritis. Nat Rev Rheumatol 2016;12(5):282–95.

49. Flagg SD, Meador R, Hsia E, et al. Decreased pain and synovial inflammation after etanercept therapy in patients with reactive and undifferentiated arthritis: an open-label trial. Arthritis Rheum 2005;53(4):613–7.

50. Meyer A, Chatelus E, Wendling D, et al. Safety and efficacy of anti-tumor necrosis factor alpha therapy in ten patients with recent-onset refractory reactive arthritis. Arthritis Rheum 2011;63(5):1274–80.

51. Wechalekar MD, Rischmueller M, Whittle S, et al. Prolonged remission of chronic reactive arthritis treated with three infusions of infliximab. J Clin Rheumatol 2010; 16(2):79–80.
52. Hannu T, Inman R, Granfors K, et al. Reactive arthritis or post-infectious arthritis? Best Pract Res Clin Rheumatol 2006;20(3):419–33.

Infections of the Spine

Maja Babic, MD[a],*, Claus S. Simpfendorfer, MD[b]

KEYWORDS

- Discitis • Spondylodiscitis • Septic facet joint • Psoas muscle abscess
- Iliacus muscle abscess

KEY POINTS

- Spine infections are on the rise in an expanding elderly population with substantial comorbidities subject to frequent invasive procedures.
- In an era of widespread use of advanced imaging modalities, the diagnostic delay of this potentially devastating condition remains unacceptably long.
- Hematogenous pyogenic septic facet joints are not a rare occurrence. They present more acutely and are frequently associated with an epidural abscess.
- Iliopsoas muscle abscess is a misnomer.
- Most psoas muscles abscesses are secondary to lumbar spondylodiscitis and can be treated conservatively if they are of musculoskeletal origin.
- Iliacus muscle abscesses are a distinct entity. They originate from a septic hip or sacroiliac joint.

INTRODUCTION

Pyogenic infections of the spine are a heterogeneous group of disorders. Most cases arise from hematogenous seeding of the axial skeleton from remote infected foci. Some are caused by direct inoculation during spinal instrumentation or contiguous spread in bedridden patients with pressure sores.[1]

The nomenclature is confusing but correlates with the underlying pathophysiology. It is presumed that the arterial route is the major pathway of hematogenous spread to the axial skeleton. In children, the nucleus pulposus of the intervertebral disc is vascularized and, therefore, susceptible to bacterial embolization, which causes a septic discitis. The abundant intraosseous arterial anastomoses seem to protect the vertebral bone from significant involvement. In the adult population, the blood vessels to the disc are obliterated, creating the largest avascular structure in the human body.

Financial Support: None.
Potential Conflicts of Interest: None.
[a] Section of Bone and Joint Infections, Department of Infectious Disease, Cleveland Clinic, 9500 Euclid Avenue, Cleveland, OH 44195, USA; [b] Section of Musculoskeletal Radiology, Imaging Institute, Cleveland Clinic, 9500 Euclid Avenue, Cleveland, OH 44195, USA
* Corresponding author.
E-mail address: babicm@ccf.org

Infect Dis Clin N Am 31 (2017) 279–297
http://dx.doi.org/10.1016/j.idc.2017.01.003
0891-5520/17/© 2017 Elsevier Inc. All rights reserved.

id.theclinics.com

However, vertebral bodies of adults have physiologic metaphyseal equivalents of long bones, which are located near the anterior longitudinal ligament and supplied by end arteriolar arcades. These are areas of slow blood flow, susceptible to bacterial seeding and subsequent occlusion promptly leading to avascular necrosis, bone infarction, and vertebral end plate osteomyelitis or spondylitis.[2] The ensuing destructive infectious process spreads into contiguous spaces, establishing a spondylodiscitis with involvement of the disc space and 2 adjacent vertebral bodies[3] (**Fig. 1**). Further spread of infection into adjoining soft tissues accounts for the development of secondary epidural abscesses, paravertebral muscle abscesses, psoas muscle abscesses (PMAs), and prevertebral collections[4] (**Figs. 2** and **3**). Occasionally, the point of hematogenous seeding of the spine can be the degenerated spinal facet joint causing a septic joint. A septic facet can extend into adjacent tissues as well, causing paraspinal muscle infections or dorsal epidural abscesses[5] (**Fig. 4**). Epidural abscesses are designated as primary exceedingly rarely nowadays (**Fig. 5**). Primary epidural abscesses account for less than 2% of all spine infections and are defined as epidural collections without contiguous infected spinal structures. Six percent of all epidural abscesses are deemed primary, whereas in 94% of cases an adjacent infected disc space or septic facet can be identified as the source of a secondary epidural abscess (**Fig. 6**).[6] Before the use of MRI as the main imaging modality for spinal infections, most epidural abscesses were deemed primary. This mostly reflects the limitations of computed tomography (CT) myelography used in the diagnosis of epidural abscesses.[7] The incidence of various manifestations of spine infections is ever changing, especially in an era of widespread use of MRI. Historically, spondylodiscitis accounted for 95% of all spine infections with 33% of cases complicated by secondary epidural abscesses, up to 6% of septic facet joints and rare cases of isolated discitis, spondylitis, and primary epidural abscesses presenting 1% to 2% percent each.[4]

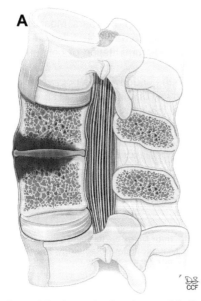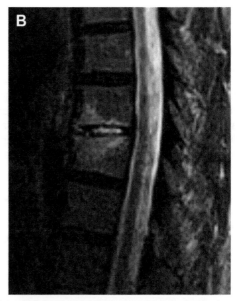

Fig. 1. (*A*) Schematic of early spondylodiscitis. (*B*) Early spondylodiscitis on sagittal MRI short tau inversion recovery (STIR) images with disc and adjacent vertebral end plate involvement. (*Courtesy of* Cleveland Clinic Foundation, Cleveland, OH; with permission.)

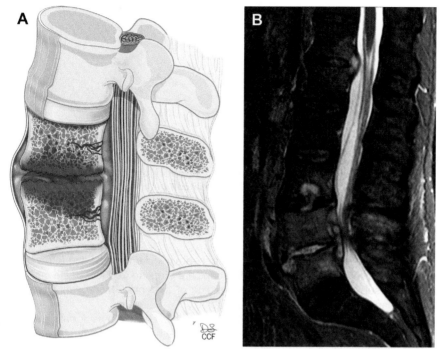

Fig. 2. (*A*) Schematic of advanced spondylodiscitis. (*B*) Advanced spondylodiscitis on sagittal MRI ST and extension of infection ventrally into prevertebral tissues. (*Courtesy of* [*A*] Cleveland Clinic Foundation, Cleveland, OH; with permission.)

Table 1 summarizes the complex spinal infection nomenclature and anatomic spread.

SPINE INFECTIONS

The incidence of spine infections in western societies is on a steady rise and has been reported to reach 6.5 cases per 100,000 each year,[8] accounting for 5% of all bone infections and representing the most frequent hematogenous osteomyelitis of the elderly.[9] The western population is aging, more patients are immunocompromised,

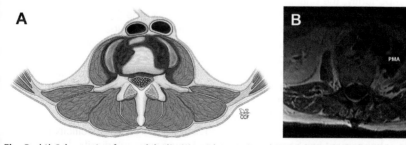

Fig. 3. (*A*) Schematic of spondylodiscitis with associated PMA. (*B*) PMA secondary to lumbar spondylodiscitis on postgadolinium T1-weighted MRI axial image. (*Courtesy of* Cleveland Clinic Foundation, Cleveland, OH; with permission.)

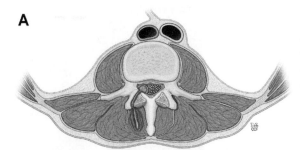
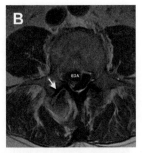

Fig. 4. (*A*) Schematic of a septic facet joint with anterior extension into epidural abscess (EDA) and posterior extension into paraspinal muscle forming an EDA and paraspinal muscle abscesses. (*B*) Septic facet joint (*arrow*) with associated EDA and paraspinal muscle abscess on postgadolinium T1-weighted MRI axial image. (*Courtesy of* Cleveland Clinic Foundation, Cleveland, OH; with permission.)

diabetic, dialysis-dependent, or with a permanent vascular access, and intravenous drug abuse is prevalent. These high-risk groups are prone to frequent bacteremic episodes and subsequent hematogenous seeding of the spine. Moreover, diagnostic tools, primarily MRI, are more readily available.

Spondylodiscitis is a challenging diagnosis to make. Back and neck pain are common complaints and routine radiographs are of little help in the early stages of the disease. Nonetheless, it is surprising that the average delay in diagnosing an infection of the spine that can lead to permanent cord injury is 2 to 4 months.[10] One should always consider spondylodiscitis in the differential of new onset back or neck pain in febrile patients, patients with endocarditis or recent gram positive bacteremia, or the previously mentioned high-risk patient groups (**Box 1**).[11] Bear in mind that fever is a common but inconsistent feature present in less than half of the patients with pyogenic spine infections and even less so in fungal, mycobacterial, and brucellar infections.[12] The back pain is located at the seeded vertebral body level and occasionally radiates to the extremities. It is exacerbated by physical activity and tends to keep patients up at night. Patients often complain that they cannot find a comfortable position in bed. Localized percussion tenderness is usually present.[13]

Box 2 lists the initial evaluation for spine infection. Inflammatory markers, such as erythrocyte sedimentation rate (ESR) and C-reactive protein (CRP), in particular, are helpful in screening for serious causes of back pain, with sensitivities greater than 95%.[14] Importantly, the only factor found to shorten the persistent diagnostic delay of pyogenic spine infection in the era of modern imaging is CRP.[15] Unfortunately, no major breakthrough has occurred over the past few decades and it still holds true that the main problem of serious spinal infections is not treatment but early diagnosis before massive neurologic symptoms occur.[16]

Secondary imaging is of paramount importance in diagnosing spondylodiscitis because it takes up to 6 weeks for bony erosive changes to manifest on plain radiography. A contrast-enhanced MRI is the imaging modality of choice.[17] The use of gadolinium is essential in differentiating between a phlegmon and a formed epidural abscess, and, if possible, should always be added.[18] It increases specificity because end plate enhancement can be the earliest sign of acute spondylodiscitis.[19] In cases in which MRI is contraindicated, contrast-enhanced CT scan, PET scan, or combined gallium/T99c bone scan can help establish the diagnosis.[20–22]

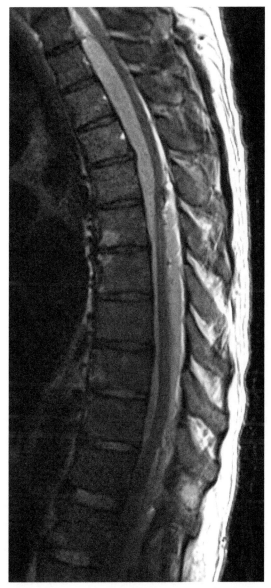

Fig. 5. Primary epidural abscess on postgadolinium T1-weighted MRI sagittal image. No spondylodiscitis or septic facet joints were found.

Blood cultures should be routinely obtained in febrile patients with back pain. They are positive in roughly 60% of bacterial spondylodiscitis cases.[23]

Every effort should be made to establish a microbiological diagnosis. Taking into account that, historically, the average delay in diagnosis lies between 2 to 4 months and that the most recent reports have not shown remarkable improvement. Empiric antibiotics should be withheld in all but critically ill patients with signs of sepsis or en route to the operating room for neurologic compromise. A CT-guided biopsy is indicated in

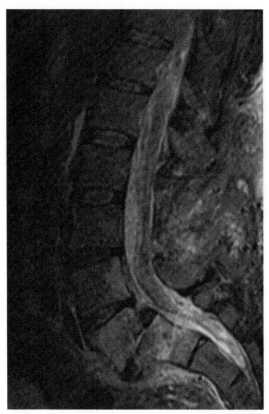

Fig. 6. Secondary epidural abscess associated with L5-S1 discitis on sagittal postgadolinium T1-weighted MRI imaging.

Table 1 Spine infection nomenclature		
Nomenclature	**Pathologic condition**	**Characteristic Features**
Discitis	Isolated disc infection	Only in vascularized discs in children
Spondylitis	Vertebral end plate infection	Very early osteomyelitis in adults
Spondylodiscitis	Disc infection with adjacent vertebral body osteomyelitis	Most spinal infections at presentation
Septic facet joint	Hematogenous pyogenic seeded septic joint	Historically rare but increasingly recognized
Primary epidural abscess	Isolated epidural abscess- no other spine element infected	Exceedingly rare in an era of MRI
Secondary epidural abscess	Contiguous spread of infection into the medullary canal	Ventral, discitis-associated Dorsal, septic facet–associated

patients with negative blood cultures or single set isolates of coagulase negative *Staphylococcus* spp in blood. The yield of biopsy ranges from 30% to 75% and is higher in cases in which empiric antibiotics have not been given.[24–26] It is deemed reasonable to withhold antibiotics up to 1 to 2 weeks in stable patients.[11] The biopsy should include an aspirate of the disc space or paravertebral soft tissue collections and a bone biopsy sample of the affected end plates. The samples are sent for both microbiology and pathohistology. Standard cultures include aerobic and anaerobic bacterial, as well as fungal stains and cultures. Mycobacterial stains and cultures are requested in cases in which exposure history and imaging findings point to possible spinal tuberculosis. Pathologic evaluation is helpful, especially in culture negative cases, in which it can confirm the presence of leukocytes, indicating pyogenic osteomyelitis or granulomas in cases of mycobacterial infection or brucellosis.[27] It can also establish an alternative diagnosis such as degenerative Modic changes, ankylosing spondylitis, hemodialysis-associated spondyloarthropathy, or neuropathic Charcot joint deformities, which present challenging imaging differentials.[28] Occasionally, crystal deposits are found on histology, primarily of the cervical spine, and aid in the diagnosis of the rare and little-known crowned dens syndrome, which can mimic spondylodiscitis but is actually a manifestation of pseudogout.[29]

Once the diagnosis is established and the microbiologic cause is confirmed, antimicrobials can be initiated (**Box 3**). Most spinal infections are treated conservatively with good outcome. It has recently been determined that 6 weeks of systemic antimicrobial therapy suffices in most cases.[30] Infections with extensive spread into paraspinal soft tissues and undrained PMAs may benefit from therapy extended to up to 8 weeks.[31] A switch to oral antibiotics with good bioavailability is acceptable once the CRP has decreased by 50%, if the pain has resolved and no residual neurologic deficits or mechanical instability are present.[3] Because most spine infections are caused by *S aureus*, it is important to reiterate that resistance to fluoroquinolones,

---

Box 3
Initial management steps for spine infection suspected or confirmed on imaging

Hemodynamically stable patient
  Hold antibiotics and plan CT-guided biopsy within 48 to 72 hours
  Empiric antibiotics following biopsy only

Hemodynamically unstable patient
  Empiric antibiotics en route to intensive care unit or meeting sepsis criteria
  Empiric antibiotics en route to operating room for reversal of neurologic deficits

---

the best oral bioavailable agents for bone infections, is on the rise and that they should not be used as monotherapy for staphylococcal spine infections.[32] The adjunct use of rifampin has been shown to be a viable alternative, though fraught with significant gastrointestinal intolerance and drug interaction issues.[33] The therapeutic response is monitored clinically and with serial inflammatory markers. Repeat cross-sectional imaging is not routinely indicated because MRI findings lag by 4 to 6 weeks. Indeed, the MRI often remains somewhat abnormal indefinitely. Only in cases in which back pain recurs and/or CRP remains persistently elevated should repeat imaging be performed.[34]

Some patients will require surgery. The indications for an operative approach include primarily symptomatic cord compression with neurologic deficits, as well as failure to control the infection with antibiotics only, in cases of unremitting back pain or prolonged bacteremia. Paralysis or motor weakness develops in 25% of patients, particularly in cases of cervical spine infections. The relapse rate of spine infection is estimated to be around 8% and the mortality of the condition remains at 6%.[23]

PYOGENIC FACET JOINT INFECTIONS

Hematogenous pyogenic facet joint infections are underappreciated and frequently overlooked. Nonetheless, they are a well-described entity with a distinct clinical picture and unique complications.

The facets, or zygapophyseal joints, are diarthrodial joints composed of opposing cartilage surfaces that interlock adjacent vertebral bodies. They contain meniscoids and are enclosed by a firm ligamentous capsule. Along with the intervertebral disc, they transfer load and constrain spine movements.[35] The loss of height of an aging intervertebral disc transfers additional weight onto the dorsal zygapophyseal joints, which are part of the 3-joint complex. The degeneration of the disc precedes the wear and tear of the respective facet joints.[36] Consequently, lumbar facet joints mirror the high risk of hematogenous seeding of their lumbar disc counterparts, followed by the cervical spine 3-joint complex. The thoracic spine, given its low shearing load, is relatively spared.

The first case of septic arthritis of a lumbar facet joint described in literature dates back to 1987, before the widespread use of MRI.[37] Herein, a 66-year-old patient presented with sudden onset of unilateral low back pain, high-grade fever and blood cultures that revealed the presence of S aureus. The notion of a normal vertebral disc at the appropriate level on plain radiography raised the possibility of infection in 1 of the numerous synovial joints of the spine. A technetium Tc99 methylene diphosphonate (MDP) bone scan showed increased uptake on the lateral aspect of L3 and L4 vertebral bodies. Eight weeks later, an end-of-treatment radiograph showed complete destruction of the right sided L3-L4 facet joint.

There is widespread belief that septic arthritis of facet joints is a rare occurrence. It has been estimated that its incidence is 500 times lower than the incidence of discitis.[38] However, Muffoletto and colleagues[5] reported an incidence of 4% (27 out of 140) of all spine infections over a 13-year period. In 2006, a Spanish study published 42 cases of septic facet joints over a 10-year period, raising its incidence to 20% of documented spine infections.[39] This echoes the experience at the authors' institution, in which the ubiquitous use of MRI as the primary imaging tool in spine infections has unveiled a more commonplace occurrence of septic facet joints than previously thought.[40] Most (>90%) cases are community-acquired, whereas a subset is iatrogenic, secondary to local facet injections or instrumentation. Cases associated with placements of epidural catheters and acupuncture have been described.[41,42] The clinical presentation of bacterial arthritis of facet joints is marked by its acuity. Patients present with sudden onset severe back pain, usually in the setting of chronic low back pain. The pain is exacerbated by flexion and extension, becomes constant, and is not relieved by rest. The delay in diagnosis from the onset of symptoms on average is less than 1 month, which is in stark contrast to the average 2 months of delay in establishing the diagnosis of spondylodiscitis.[43,44] Unlike in cases of spondylodiscitis, patients can usually determine the laterality of the back pain.[45] Radicular symptoms with pain radiating to the flank or buttock are reported in half the cases. Exquisite palpatory tenderness of the ipsilateral paraspinal musculature is present. Unlike the average spondylodiscitis cases, patients with a seeded septic facet joint are more likely to be febrile (>80%). Neurologic deficits can be marked on presentation.[5]

Predisposing factors seem to be the same risk factors that lead to spondylodiscitis. They correlate with a higher incidence of transient bacteremic episodes in a patient population with degenerative disc disease and facet arthropathy, and include primarily diabetes, chronic kidney disorders, liver disease, immunosuppression, and intravenous substance abuse. The presence of a chronic vascular access, indwelling dialysis catheters, and frequent skin barrier breaches present entry portals for organisms that can seed both the end arterial arcades of vertebral bodies and facet joints.

Historically, it was thought that posterior element involvement was unusual in pyogenic spine infections and most cases were attributed to neoplasm, coccidioidomycosis, and actinomycosis.[44] It has since been established that, as in spondylodiscitis, the most frequently isolated organism is S aureus.[46] In contrast to spondylodiscitis though, and probably due to its more acute presentation, the causative organism is found in most cases, with the yield of aspirates and tissue cultures of over 75% and combined blood culture and aspirate yields in greater than 90% of cases.[5] Needle aspiration under CT guidance in cases that are not associated with bacteremia are frequently diagnostic and provide therapeutic relief.[47,48]

Imaging is of pivotal importance in establishing the diagnosis. A high index of suspicion is needed. Plain radiographs as the initial screen for sudden onset back pain are of little help in the acute setting. The findings lag 6 to 12 weeks and display erosive changes, including irregular facet joints, pseudo enlargement of the joints, or joint space narrowing.[37,49] The use of nuclear scans was prevalent in the past decade and both Tc99 MDP and gallium-67 scintigraphy showed uptake in affected facets, indicating inflammatory changes early in the course of the disease.[50,51]

In contrast, CT imaging findings lag by 2 weeks but demonstrate erosive changes in affected facets, as well as additional soft tissue spread, and can delineate the extent of involvement of the epidural space, paraspinal, or psoas musculature.[52,53] Importantly, CT is the primary imaging modality used for guided aspirations, soft tissue biopsy, and therapeutic decompression of the septic facet.

With the advancement and widespread availability of MRI, these modalities have mostly become alternative choices, save for cases in which the use of a magnetic field is contraindicated. MRI images demonstrate joint space destruction and intraarticular fluid on T2-weighted images, as well as enhancement of surrounding tissues, epidural, paraspinal, or psoas muscle phlegmon or abscesses on postgadoliniumT1-weighted images. It is a very sensitive and specific imaging modality for septic facet joints, and can be used to demonstrate changes very early on.[54] It can establish the diagnosis as early as 5 days following onset of back pain.[55]

The optimal therapeutic approach to septic facet joints has yet to be elucidated. As in the case of spondylodiscitis, the pathogenesis is believed to be hematogenous seeding of facet joints that are already afflicted by degenerative joint changes.[56] Terminal branches of the lumbar arteries provide blood flow to the facet joints, paraspinal muscles, and posterior epidural space. It is important to mention that infections of the septic facet can be associated with extension into the epidural space. The frequency of a septic facet with concomitant epidural abscess varies between series but has been recorded to be anywhere between 25% and 60% of cases.[5,39,56] Given the lack of consensus in the treatment of septic facet joints, most are treated according to vertebral osteomyelitis guidelines. Most cases rely on medical therapy. Antibiotics are administered on average for 6 weeks intravenously or until inflammatory markers normalize.[11] Aspiration under CT guidance of purulent content from the facet joint helps with faster relief of symptoms but most cases are treated conservatively.[5,57] Surgical debridement is necessary in cases of clinical failure, persistent pain, ongoing bacteremia, or neurologic deficits. It seems that cervical septic facets undergo surgical management in most cases because extension into the epidural space frequently manifests with neurologic deficits.[58] Cases associated with steroid injections of facet joints also tend to require decompression more frequently and present more acutely within days following the injection.[59,60]

In summary, the widespread use of MRI has raised awareness of septic facet arthritis in an era of aging population, advanced degenerative spinal joint disease, and ever-growing medical instrumentation. It is an entity that has overlapping features of septic arthritis of large cartilaginous joints and spondylodiscitis. It classically presents with acute unilateral back pain in a febrile patient. It is associated with bacteremia more often than spondylodiscitis. Epidural extension is frequent. Most cases can be treated conservatively. Surgery is required in most cervical septic facets, steroid injection–related septic facets, and all that progress to neurologic deficits, persistent pain, and ongoing bacteremia.

The key differences between discitis and septic facet joint are summarized in **Table 2**.

Curious entities associated with septic facet joints that are rarely encountered and frequently overlooked are septic costovertebral and costotransverse joints (**Fig. 7**).

Table 2
Distinguishing features of septic facet joints versus spondylodiscitis

Entity	Cause Hematogenous Seeding	Onset	Fever	Diagnostic Delay	Location of Pain	Secondary Epidural Abscess
Septic facet joint	Yes	Acute	++	<4 wk	Unilateral	Up to 60%
Spondylodiscitis	Yes	Subacute	+	2–4 mo	Midline	Up to 30%

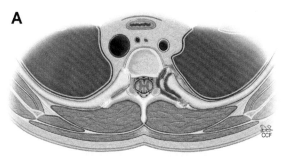 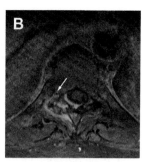

Fig. 7. (*A*) Schematic of a septic costovertebral-transverse joint. (*B*) Postgadolinium T1-weighted MRI image of a septic costotransverse and infected costovertebral joint (*arrow*) associated with an ipsilateral septic facet and epidural abscess. (*Courtesy of* Cleveland Clinic Foundation, Cleveland, OH; with permission.)

The costovertebral joint is the articulation between the vertebral body and the head of the rib, whereas the costotransverse joint is the articulation between the rib and the transverse process of the thoracic vertebrae.[61] Occasionally, the infectious process can extend from an adjacent septic facet and engulf the articulations between the thoracic vertebrae and the rib. This accounts for a rather unconventional clinical presentation. Patients can present with unilateral chest pain, pain radiating into the scapula or the sternum, or pain extending along the rib, exacerbated by movement and inspiration, and can, therefore, be mistaken for either pleuritic chest pain or herpes zoster.

SPONDYLODISCITIS AND PSOAS MUSCLE ABSCESS

The iliopsoas muscle is the major hip flexor and is comprised of 2 distinct muscles, the psoas and the iliacus muscle, that share a tendon attachment site on the lesser trochanter. Conventional surgical terminology does not differentiate between abscesses located in the iliacus or psoas muscle, yet the causes, clinical picture, and outcomes differ significantly.[62] The term iliopsoas muscle is, therefore, somewhat of a misnomer.[61]

The psoas muscle attaches proximally at the lateral side and transverse processes of the lumbar vertebrae and corresponding intervertebral discs (T12-L5). It joins the tendon of the iliacus muscle below the inguinal ligament and attaches distally to the lesser trochanter. The blood supply to the psoas muscle stems from branches of the lumbar arteries and includes a rich venous communication with the paravertebral lumbar plexus. The origin of the iliacus muscle is formed by the hollow iliac fossa, the upper sacrum, and the sacroiliac (SI) and iliolumbar ligaments between them. Each muscle is enveloped in its respective fascia. The bottom of the iliac fossa, between the psoas and iliacus muscle, is occupied by a conjoined bursa, the bulk of which lies under the iliacus muscle.[61] The iliopsoas bursa is the largest bursa in the human body, present in 98% of the population. It lies anterior to the hip joint with which it communicates in 15% of asymptomatic individuals.[63] Following placement of a prosthetic hip, the postoperative joint capsule can communicate with the iliopsoas bursa with increasing frequency.[64] The communication between the bursa and the hip joint is of paramount clinical importance, especially in patients with inflammatory disorders and prosthetic hip implants because it presents the path of least resistance for pathologic processes, primarily infections.

Historically, iliopsoas muscle abscess (IPA) has been deemed a rare clinical entity.[65] In the 1980s, a retrospective study of more than 300 cases spanning a century from 1881 to 1985 estimated a rate of 3 cases per year in a single tertiary center.[66] More recent studies from England and Spain showed an increase in the number of annual cases but still consider the entity an uncommon.[67,68] The authors believe it is likely due to underreporting because the widespread use of cross-sectional imaging has improved diagnostic accuracy significantly.

Traditionally, IPA has been classified as primary if no adjacent anatomic structure could be identified as the source of infection. Primary abscesses were thought to arise from hematogenous seeding of a bruised muscle and were more frequent in younger, active, male patients. Of note, primary abscess reports came mostly out of Asia and Africa, where the bulk (99.5%) of IPA were deemed primary.[69] Abscesses classified as secondary occur by direct spread from adjacent structures.

The most frequent cause of secondary IPA listed in medical literature continues to be intraabdominal disease, despite newer case series implicating that most cases are related to skeletal infectious sources.[67,70–72] The root of this bias likely stems from the original case series in the 1980s when all patients with diagnosed IPA were treated at a tertiary center for inflammatory bowel disease.[65,73] Most cases of IPA were diagnosed intraoperatively and drained as part of an attempt to control fistulizing Crohn disease.

Newer data emphasize that abscesses in the iliopsoas compartment most frequently arise from adjacent skeletal structures. PMAs are most frequently secondary to spondylodiscitis of the lumbar spine.[67] Iliacus muscle abscesses (IMAs) are caused by spread of infection from the SI joint or the hip.[62]

Given these gradations of pathophysiology, the authors prefer to refer to them as distinct entities and avoid the misnomer IPA.

The PMA is referred to as a disease in evolution and its microbiology has been in flux.[74] Since the original description by Herman Mynter in 1881[75], the microbiology has vastly changed. During the early twentieth century, most cases were attributed to *Mycobacterium tuberculosis*. Mirroring the evolution of vertebral osteomyelitis, *M tuberculosis* as the predominant organism has largely been replaced by *S aureus*.[71,76] Most IMA at present are also caused by *S aureus*.[62]

Patients with lumbar spine spondylodiscitis and secondary PMA can present with back pain and hip pain. They are frequently febrile.[71] Few patients present with the full psoas abscess triad with fever, back pain, and a limp. The presentation of an IMA is more varied but mostly includes hip pain or buttock pain.[62,77]

In most cases, inflammatory markers, including the CRP and ESR, are elevated. Blood cultures can be positive. In a recent case series this was so in more than 40% of cases.[71] These data, however, do not differentiate between PMA and IMA because most published series lump these 2 entities together.

Cross-sectional imaging is crucial in establishing the diagnosis. Plain films that are routinely ordered in the workup of back pain are rather insensitive, both for diagnosing changes of vertebral osteomyelitis as well as the secondary PMAs associated with it. A failure to visualize the lateral margin of the psoas muscle on supine abdominal films indicates a retroperitoneal pathologic condition, including PMA, and is labeled as the radiographic psoas sign.[78] On MRI, the psoas sign is known as the look-at-me lesion. The hyperintense changes on T2-weighted images in the psoas muscle correlate highly with lumbar spondylodiscitis and improve diagnostic accuracy on MRI.[79] PMAs are diagnosed coincidentally by contrast-enhanced MRI in patients suspected of harboring an infection in the spine. They can be either unilateral or bilateral, and are frequently multiloculated. They are adjacent to infected disc spaces, vertebral bodies, or septic facets of the lumbar spine because the psoas muscle attaches proximally to the lumbar transverse processes. On CT imaging, PMA present as asymmetric enlargement of the muscle by a lesion of low attenuation (**Fig. 8**). They are seen as well-delineated hypodense collections with a bright rim on contrast-enhanced studies, both CT and MRI.[68] CT is the main imaging modality used for guided percutaneous aspiration. Nuclear imaging is occasionally used but has fallen out of favor since the advent of MRI, mainly due to its lower sensitivity and overall poor spatial resolution. Nonetheless, in patients who have implantable devices, such as defibrillators, cochlear implants, or remnant metal bullets, in proximity to vital structures, the clinician can resort to nuclear imaging to establish a diagnosis of lumbar spondylodiscitis and secondary PMA. IMAs are diagnosed coincidentally as well on CT scans and MRIs ordered for hip or buttock pain or pain in the SI joint. The IMA presents as a hypodense collection on CT, with an enhancing rim if contrast is used. The iliacus muscle is asymmetrically enlarged on 1 side and, depending on the duration of symptoms, erosive changes can be seen in the ipsilateral SI joint. On MRI, unilateral fluid in the SI joint is present with concomitant edema in the bone, elucidating the origin of the collection in the iliacus muscle secondary to pyogenic sacroiliitis.[80] Plain radiography and ultrasound are of limited use. Nuclear scans, as in cases of lumbar spondylodiscitis or PMA, can occasionally be used in selected cases but lack spatial resolution and cannot determine the anatomic origin of the IMA.

The diagnosis of IMA associated with an infected native or prosthetic hip joints presents a considerable clinical challenge. Because cross-sectional imaging is not part of a routine workup for suspected infected hip joints, collections in the iliacus muscle

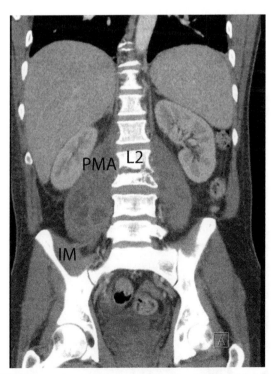

Fig. 8. Coronal CT images contrast-enhanced of multiloculated right-sided PMAs secondary to L2-3 spondylodiscitis. IM, iliacus muscle.

associated with septic hips are frequently missed. Plain radiographs can demonstrate periprosthetic lucencies, periosteal thickening, and extensive heterotopic bone formation, raising suspicion for underlying prosthetic joint infection and prompting a diagnostic hip aspiration. Diagnostic contrast injection can occasionally demonstrate extravasation of the contrast beyond the hip joint into the pelvic space. A definitive diagnosis of an IMA is made only with the help of cross-sectional imaging, either CT or MRI. A high degree of clinical suspicion is needed and, unfortunately, IMA can go unnoticed until several prosthetic joint revisions have failed. It has been recommended that hematogenously seeded prosthetic hip infections undergo CT scanning to detect cases with extension of infection into the adjacent iliac muscle[81] (**Fig. 9**).

Management of PMA and IMA differ. Historically, PMA drainage was considered standard of therapy but no clear preference was given to open surgical versus percutaneous drainage.[82–85] More recent reports favor less invasive methods, including conservative management with antibiotics only.[86] It has been suggested that larger PMAs with a cut-off greater than 3 cm in diameter should be drained percutaneously and that smaller collections can be managed conservatively with antibiotics only. This, however, is an arbitrary cut-off imposed by technical limitations because cavities less than 3 cm in diameter present insufficient space for exchange of wires, dilators, and the formation of the distal loop of the drainage catheter.[87] Successful conservative management, with antimicrobial therapy only, of collections ranging from 2.5 to 7.5 cm has been reported.[88] In the authors' experience, PMA secondary to lumbar spondylodiscitis will resolve without drainage over the 6-week course of standard antibiotic therapy given for vertebral osteomyelitis. At the authors' institution, CT-guided aspiration of PMA is done mainly for diagnostic purposes in spondylodiscitis cases with negative blood cultures at 48 hours.

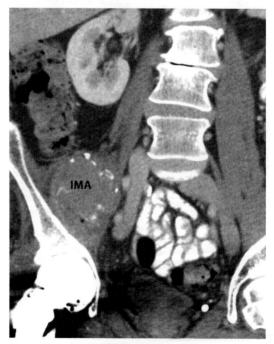

Fig. 9. IMA secondary to a septic hip joint.

IMAs are managed differently and seem to have a less favorable prognosis. Cases associated with septic sacroiliitis usually resolve with extended antibiotic therapy because surgical management of the partially syndesmotic joint is rarely undertaken.[89] In general, a 6-week course of targeted antibiotic treatment is suggested. The approach to IMA secondary to an infected prosthetic hip joint has not been standardized. It always involves revision of the infected hip but whether open drainage through an anterior approach offers a therapeutic advantage has yet to be determined.

In summary, PMA are most frequently secondary to lumbar spondylodiscitis. They are often an incidental finding and do not require surgical management if they are of musculoskeletal origin. CT-guided aspiration is recommended for diagnostic purposes. Most will resolve with conservative antibiotic treatment of the spondylodiscitis without percutaneous drainage.

REFERENCES

1. Friedman JA, Maher CO, Quast LM, et al. Spontaneous disc space infections in adults. Surg Neurol 2002;57(2):81–6.
2. Govender S. Spinal infections. J Bone Joint Surg Br 2005;87(11):1454–8.
3. Lam KS, Webb JK. Discitis. Hosp Med 2004;65(5):280–6.
4. Hadjipavlou AG, Mader JT, Necessary JT, et al. Hematogenous pyogenic spinal infections and their surgical management. Spine (Phila Pa 1976) 2000;25(13): 1668–79.
5. Muffoletto AJ, Ketonen LM, Mader JT, et al. Hematogenous pyogenic facet joint infection. Spine (Phila Pa 1976) 2001;26(14):1570–6.
6. Hadjipavlou AG, Berguist S, Chen J, et al. Vertebral osteomyelitis. Cur Treat Options 2000;2:226–37.
7. Reihsaus E, Waldbaur H, Seeling W. Spinal epidural abscess: a meta-analysis of 915 patients. Neurosurg Rev 2000;23(4):175–204 [discussion: 205].
8. Grammatico L, Baron S, Rusch E, et al. Epidemiology of vertebral osteomyelitis (VO) in France: analysis of hospital-discharge data 2002-2003. Epidemiol Infect 2008;136(5):653–60.
9. Jensen AG, Espersen F, Skinhoj P, et al. Increasing frequency of vertebral osteomyelitis following *Staphylococcus aureus* bacteraemia in Denmark 1980-1990. J Infect 1997;34(2):113–8.
10. Gasbarrini AL, Bertoldi E, Mazzetti M, et al. Clinical features, diagnostic and therapeutic approaches to haematogenous vertebral osteomyelitis. Eur Rev Med Pharmacol Sci 2005;9(1):53–66.
11. Berbari EF, Kanj SS, Kowalski TJ, et al. 2015 Infectious Diseases Society of America (IDSA) clinical practice guidelines for the diagnosis and treatment of native vertebral osteomyelitis in adults. Clin Infect Dis 2015;61(6):e26–46.
12. Mrabet D, Mizouni H, Khiari H, et al. Brucellar spondylodiscitis affecting noncontiguous spine levels. BMJ Case Rep 2011;2011.
13. McHenry MC, Easley KA, Locker GA. Vertebral osteomyelitis: long-term outcome for 253 patients from 7 Cleveland-area hospitals. Clin Infect Dis 2002;34(10): 1342–50.
14. Siemionow K, Steinmetz M, Bell G, et al. Identifying serious causes of back pain: cancer, infection, fracture. Cleve Clin J Med 2008;75(8):557–66.
15. Jean M, Irisson JO, Gras G, et al. Diagnostic delay of pyogenic vertebral osteomyelitis and its associated factors. Scand J Rheumatol 2017;46(1):64–8.
16. Strohecker J, Grobovschek M. Spinal epidural abscess: an interdisciplinary emergency. Zentralbl Neurochir 1986;47(2):120–4 [in German].

17. Dagirmanjian A, Schils J, McHenry M, et al. MR imaging of vertebral osteomyelitis revisited. AJR Am J Roentgenol 1996;167(6):1539–43.
18. Ledermann HP, Schweitzer ME, Morrison WB, et al. MR imaging findings in spinal infections: rules or myths? Radiology 2003;228(2):506–14.
19. Dunbar JA, Sandoe JA, Rao AS, et al. The MRI appearances of early vertebral osteomyelitis and discitis. Clin Radiol 2010;65(12):974–81.
20. Palestro CJ, Torres MA. Radionuclide imaging in orthopedic infections. Semin Nucl Med 1997;27(4):334–45.
21. Love C, Patel M, Lonner BS, et al. Diagnosing spinal osteomyelitis: a comparison of bone and Ga-67 scintigraphy and magnetic resonance imaging. Clin Nucl Med 2000;25(12):963–77.
22. Ohtori S, Suzuki M, Koshi T, et al. 18F-fluorodeoxyglucose-PET for patients with suspected spondylitis showing Modic change. Spine (Phila Pa 1976) 2010; 35(26):E1599–603.
23. Mylona E, Samarkos M, Kakalou E, et al. Pyogenic vertebral osteomyelitis: a systematic review of clinical characteristics. Semin Arthritis Rheum 2009;39(1):10–7.
24. de Lucas EM, Gonzalez Mandly A, Gutierrez A, et al. CT-guided fine-needle aspiration in vertebral osteomyelitis: true usefulness of a common practice. Clin Rheumatol 2009;28(3):315–20.
25. Kim CJ, Song KH, Park WB, et al. Microbiologically and clinically diagnosed vertebral osteomyelitis: impact of prior antibiotic exposure. Antimicrob Agents Chemother 2012;56(4):2122–4.
26. Rankine JJ, Barron DA, Robinson P, et al. Therapeutic impact of percutaneous spinal biopsy in spinal infection. Postgrad Med J 2004;80(948):607–9.
27. Zimmerli W. Clinical practice. Vertebral osteomyelitis. N Engl J Med 2010; 362(11):1022–9.
28. Hong SH, Choi JY, Lee JW, et al. MR imaging assessment of the spine: infection or an imitation? Radiographics 2009;29(2):599–612.
29. Godfrin-Valnet M, Godfrin G, Godard J, et al. Eighteen cases of crowned dens syndrome: presentation and diagnosis. Neurochirurgie 2013;59(3):115–20.
30. Bernard L, Dinh A, Ghout I, et al. Antibiotic treatment for 6 weeks versus 12 weeks in patients with pyogenic vertebral osteomyelitis: an open-label, non-inferiority, randomised, controlled trial. Lancet 2015;385(9971):875–82.
31. Park KH, Cho OH, Lee JH, et al. Optimal duration of antibiotic therapy in patients with hematogenous vertebral osteomyelitis at low risk and high risk of recurrence. Clin Infect Dis 2016;62(10):1262–9.
32. Coskun-Ari FF, Bosgelmez-Tinaz G. grlA and gyrA mutations and antimicrobial susceptibility in clinical isolates of ciprofloxacin- methicillin-resistant Staphylococcus aureus. Eur J Med Res 2008;13(8):366–70.
33. Schrenzel J, Harbarth S, Schockmel G, et al. A randomized clinical trial to compare fleroxacin-rifampicin with flucloxacillin or vancomycin for the treatment of staphylococcal infection. Clin Infect Dis 2004;39(9):1285–92.
34. Kowalski TJ, Berbari EF, Huddleston PM, et al. Do follow-up imaging examinations provide useful prognostic information in patients with spine infection? Clin Infect Dis 2006;43(2):172–9.
35. Jaumard NV, Welch WC, Winkelstein BA. Spinal facet joint biomechanics and mechanotransduction in normal, injury and degenerative conditions. J Biomech Eng 2011;133(7):071010.
36. Yong-Hing K, Kirkaldy-Willis WH. The pathophysiology of degenerative disease of the lumbar spine. Orthop Clin North Am 1983;14(3):491–504.

37. Halpin DS, Gibson RD. Septic arthritis of a lumbar facet joint. J Bone Joint Surg Br 1987;69(3):457–9.

38. David-Chausse J, Dehais J, Boyer M, et al. Articular infections in adults. Peripheral and vertebral involvement with common bacteria and tubercle bacteria. Rev Rhum Mal Osteoartic 1981;48(1):69–76 [in French].

39. Narvaez J, Nolla JM, Narvaez JA, et al. Spontaneous pyogenic facet joint infection. Semin Arthritis Rheum 2006;35(5):272–83.

40. Diehn FE. Imaging of spine infection. Radiol Clin North Am 2012;50(4):777–98.

41. Peris P, Brancos MA, Gratacos J, et al. Septic arthritis of spinal apophyseal joint. Report of two cases and review of the literature. Spine (Phila Pa 1976) 1992; 17(12):1514–6.

42. Glaser JA, El-Khoury GY. Unknown case. Diagnosis: facet joint septic arthritis T12-L1 on the left with extension of the infection into the spinal canal producing a large epidural abscess. Spine (Phila Pa 1976) 2001;26(8):991–3.

43. Nolla JM, Ariza J, Gomez-Vaquero C, et al. Spontaneous pyogenic vertebral osteomyelitis in nondrug users. Semin Arthritis Rheum 2002;31(4):271–8.

44. Sapico FL, Montgomerie JZ. Vertebral osteomyelitis. Infect Dis Clin North Am 1990;4(3):539–50.

45. Masson C, Laffite A, Audran M. Arthritis septique de l'articulation interapophysaire posterieure du rachis. Rev Rhum Mal Osteoartic 2006;73:369–72.

46. Michel-Batot C, Dintinger H, Blum A, et al. A particular form of septic arthritis: septic arthritis of facet joint. Joint Bone Spine 2008;75(1):78–83.

47. Ben Hamouda M, Rajhi H, Golli M, et al. Septic arthritis of posterior lumbar facet joint. J Radiol 1997;78(5):373–6 [in French].

48. Rousselin B, Gires F, Vallee C, et al. Case report 627: septic arthritis of lumbar facet joint as initial manifestation of spondylodiscitis. Skeletal Radiol 1990; 19(6):453–5.

49. Roberts WA. Pyogenic vertebral osteomyelitis of a lumbar facet joint with associated epidural abscess. A case report with review of the literature. Spine (Phila Pa 1976) 1988;13(8):948–52.

50. Hadjipavlou AG, Cesani-Vazquez F, Villaneuva-Meyer J, et al. The effectiveness of gallium citrate Ga 67 radionuclide imaging in vertebral osteomyelitis revisited. Am J Orthop (Belle Mead NJ) 1998;27(3):179–83.

51. Swayne LC, Dorsky S, Caruana V, et al. Septic arthritis of a lumbar facet joint: detection with bone SPECT imaging. J Nucl Med 1989;30(8):1408–11.

52. Tay BK, Deckey J, Hu SS. Spinal infections. J Am Acad Orthop Surg 2002;10(3): 188–97.

53. Tali ET, Gultekin S. Spinal infections. Eur Radiol 2005;15(3):599–607.

54. Pilleul F, Garcia J. Septic arthritis of the spine facet joint: early positive diagnosis on magnetic resonance imaging. Review of two cases. Joint Bone Spine 2000; 67(3):234–7.

55. Andre V, Pot-Vaucel M, Cozic C, et al. Septic arthritis of the facet joint. Med Mal Infect 2015;45(6):215–21.

56. Ergan M, Macro M, Benhamou CL, et al. Septic arthritis of lumbar facet joints. A review of six cases. Rev Rhum Engl Ed 1997;64(6):386–95.

57. Doita M, Nabeshima Y, Nishida K, et al. Septic arthritis of lumbar facet joints without predisposing infection. J Spinal Disord Tech 2007;20(4):290–5.

58. Stecher JM, El-Khoury GY, Hitchon PW. Cervical facet joint septic arthritis: a case report. Iowa Orthop J 2010;30:182–7.

59. Weingarten TN, Hooten WM, Huntoon MA. Septic facet joint arthritis after a corticosteroid facet injection. Pain Med 2006;7(1):52–6.

60. Compes P, Rakotozanany P, Dufour H, et al. Spontaneous atlantoaxial pyogenic arthritis surgically managed. Eur Spine J 2015;24(Suppl 4):S461–4.
61. McDonald SW. Last's anatomy: regional and applied. 8th edition. London: Churchill Livingstone; 1991.
62. Shyam Kumar AJ, Hickerton B, Smith IC, et al. Iliacus abscess: an entity to be differentiated from psoas abscess: a review of 15 cases. Eur J Orthop Surg Traumatol 2007;17:477–8.
63. Allen WC, Cope R. Coxa saltans: the snapping hip revisited. J Am Acad Orthop Surg 1995;3(5):303–8.
64. Steinbach LS, Schneider R, Goldman AB, et al. Bursae and abscess cavities communicating with the hip. Diagnosis using arthrography and CT. Radiology 1985;156(2):303–7.
65. Ricci MA, Rose FB, Meyer KK. Pyogenic psoas abscess: worldwide variations in etiology. World J Surg 1986;10(5):834–43.
66. Bartolo DC, Ebbs SR, Cooper MJ. Psoas abscess in Bristol: a 10-year review. Int J Colorectal Dis 1987;2(2):72–6.
67. Navarro Lopez V, Ramos JM, Meseguer V, et al. Microbiology and outcome of iliopsoas abscess in 124 patients. Medicine (Baltimore) 2009;88(2):120–30.
68. Torres GM, Cernigliaro JG, Abbitt PL, et al. Iliopsoas compartment: normal anatomy and pathologic processes. Radiographics 1995;15(6):1285–97.
69. Desandre AR, Cottone FJ, Evers ML. Iliopsoas abscess: etiology, diagnosis, and treatment. Am Surg 1995;61(12):1087–91.
70. Muckley T, Schutz T, Hierholzer C, et al. Psoas abscess after anterior spinal fusion. Unfallchirurg 2003;106(3):252–8 [in German].
71. Alonso CD, Barclay S, Tao X, et al. Increasing incidence of iliopsoas abscesses with MRSA as a predominant pathogen. J Infect 2011;63(1):1–7.
72. Dietrich A, Vaccarezza H, Vaccaro CA. Iliopsoas abscess: presentation, management, and outcomes. Surg Laparosc Endosc Percutan Tech 2013;23(1):45–8.
73. Procaccino JA, Lavery IC, Fazio VW, et al. Psoas abscess: difficulties encountered. Dis Colon Rectum 1991;34(9):784–9.
74. Franco-Paredes C, Blumberg HM. Psoas muscle abscess caused by Mycobacterium tuberculosis and Staphylococcus aureus: case report and review. Am J Med Sci 2001;321(6):415–7.
75. Mynter H. Acute psoitis. Buffalo Med Surg 1881:J21-202.
76. Gordin F, Stamler C, Mills J. Pyogenic psoas abscesses: noninvasive diagnostic techniques and review of the literature. Rev Infect Dis 1983;5(6):1003–11.
77. Simons GW, Sty JR, Starshak RR. Iliacus abscess. Clin Orthop Relat Res 1984;(183):61–3.
78. Williams SM, Harned RK, Hultman SA, et al. The psoas sign: a reevaluation. Radiographics 1985;5:525–36.
79. Ledbetter LN, Salzman KL, Shah LM. Imaging psoas sign in lumbar spinal infections: evaluation of diagnostic accuracy and comparison with established imaging characteristics. AJNR Am J Neuroradiol 2016;37(4):736–41.
80. Sandrasegaran K, Saifuddin A, Coral A, et al. Magnetic resonance imaging of septic sacroiliitis. Skeletal Radiol 1994;23(4):289–92.
81. Dauchy FA, Dupon M, Dutronc H, et al. Association between psoas abscess and prosthetic hip infection: a case-control study. Acta Orthop 2009;80(2):198–200.
82. McAuliffe W, Clarke G. The diagnosis and treatment of psoas abscess: a 12 year review. Aust N Z J Surg 1994;64(6):413–7.
83. Gupta S, Suri S, Gulati M, et al. Ilio-psoas abscesses: percutaneous drainage under image guidance. Clin Radiol 1997;52(9):704–7.

84. Cantasdemir M, Kara B, Cebi D, et al. Computed tomography-guided percutaneous catheter drainage of primary and secondary iliopsoas abscesses. Clin Radiol 2003;58(10):811–5.

85. Baier PK, Arampatzis G, Imdahl A, et al. The iliopsoas abscess: aetiology, therapy, and outcome. Langenbecks Arch Surg 2006;391(4):411–7.

86. Yacoub WN, Sohn HJ, Chan S, et al. Psoas abscess rarely requires surgical intervention. Am J Surg 2008;196(2):223–7.

87. Charles HW. Abscess drainage. Semin Intervent Radiol 2012;29(4):325–36.

88. van den Berge M, de Marie S, Kuipers T, et al. Psoas abscess: report of a series and review of the literature. Neth J Med 2005;63(10):413–6.

89. Osman AA, Govender S. Septic sacroiliitis. Clin Orthop Relat Res 1995;(313): 214–9.

Radiologic Approach to Musculoskeletal Infections

Claus S. Simpfendorfer, MD

KEYWORDS

- Musculoskeletal infections • Necrotizing fasciitis • Periprosthetic joint infection
- Osteomyelitis • Spondylodiscitis • Septic facet joint • MRI

KEY POINTS

- Conventional radiography should always be the first imaging examination performed in all suspected musculoskeletal infections.
- Normal radiographs should not delay further diagnostic workup with cross-sectional imaging in suspected musculoskeletal infections.
- Aspiration should be performed after radiographs on all suspected cases of periprosthetic joint infection, septic arthritis, bursitis, and tenosynovitis.
- MRI, which can evaluate both bone and soft tissue, is the preferred imaging examination for diagnosis and evaluation of soft tissue infections, spine infections, and osteomyelitis.
- Intravenous gadolinium should be administered when performing MRI in all suspected musculoskeletal infections unless contraindicated.

INTRODUCTION

Approximately 2 million patients are treated annually within the United States for musculoskeletal infections.[1] Imaging is often used to establish a diagnosis and evaluate the full extent and severity of disease, ultimately impacting treatment. Although often nondiagnostic, imaging should always start with radiographs, which provide an important anatomic overview and can impact both the choice and interpretation of the subsequent advanced imaging examination. MRI is the test of choice in most musculoskeletal infections secondary to its superior soft tissue contrast resolution and high sensitivity for pathologic fluid.[2-4] However, MRI is not always available and when available may not be possible secondary to multiple contraindicated implanted devices or severe claustrophobia. Alternative imaging modalities including ultrasound scan, computed tomography (CT), and radionuclide imaging may be used. This article reviews the individual imaging modalities including how and when they should be used

Financial Support: None.
Potential Conflicts of Interest: None.
Section of Musculoskeletal Radiology, Imaging Institute, Cleveland Clinic, CCLCM/CWRU, 9500 Euclid Avenue, Cleveland, OH 44195, USA
E-mail address: simpfec2@ccf.org

Infect Dis Clin N Am 31 (2017) 299–324
http://dx.doi.org/10.1016/j.idc.2017.01.004
0891-5520/17/© 2017 Elsevier Inc. All rights reserved.

id.theclinics.com

and discusses specific musculoskeletal infections and how they should be approached from an imaging perspective.

CONVENTIONAL RADIOGRAPHS

Radiographs should be the first imaging examination performed for all suspected musculoskeletal infections. Whether as an outpatient or inpatient or in an emergency setting, radiographs are readily available and inexpensive. Although radiographs are typically nondiagnostic early in the disease process, they aid in the selection and interpretation of follow-up cross-sectional imaging.[5]

COMPUTED TOMOGRAPHY

CT has a high spatial resolution providing the best bony detail of all the imaging modalities and can detect changes of osteomyelitis earlier than conventional radiographs. The superior evaluation of the osseous structures makes CT the best imaging modality for identifying the sequestra, cloacae, or involucra associated with chronic osteomyelitis.[5] CT has the added value of being able to evaluate the surrounding soft tissues and provide detailed analysis of compartmental anatomy. Evaluation of the soft tissues is improved with the use of intravenous contrast, allowing better depiction of fluid collections, joint effusions, and soft tissue inflammation. Furthermore, the ability of CT to survey a large area in a very short time makes it the cross-sectional test of choice in emergency departments.[1] CT remains less desirable than MRI because of decreased soft tissue contrast and inability to detect early changes of osteomyelitis. Additional disadvantages of CT include its use of ionizing radiation and degraded images secondary to metallic artifact.

ULTRASOUND SCAN

Ultrasound scan is typically used when evaluating fluid collections, such as a soft tissue abscess or joint effusion. Aspiration can then be performed under ultrasound guidance when needed. Ultrasound scan can be used for acute osteomyelitis in the pediatric population by identifying a subperiosteal abscess and guiding aspiration.[6] The benefit of ultrasound scan in the pediatric population is that it can be rapidly performed, does not require sedation, and does not use ionizing radiation. However, ultrasound scan is operator dependent and of little value in adult osteomyelitis because of its inability to penetrate the cortex of the bone.

RADIONUCLIDE IMAGING

Radionuclide imaging is the most confusing and nuanced imaging modality, with multiple different examinations and radiopharmaceuticals, which can be combined to improve accuracy. All examinations are plagued by low spatial resolution, which can be improved by the use of single-photon emission computed tomography (SPECT) or preferably integrated SPECT-CT. Likewise, the utility of PET imaging has also increased with the introduction of combined PET-CT. This article reviews the most commonly used and available of these examinations.

THREE-PHASE BONE SCINTIGRAPHY

Bone scintigraphy is performed with technetium-99m (^{99m}Tc)-labeled diphosphonates. The 3 phases include a blood flow, blood pool, and delayed bone phases. The test is completed in 2 to 4 hours and is extremely sensitive for osteomyelitis.

The test, however, is not specific, and multiple etiologies affecting bone turnover including infection, recent surgery, orthopedic hardware, and neuropathic joints can result in a positive scan.[7,8] Bone scintigraphy is most effective when evaluating non-violated bone or when used as a screening examination for periprosthetic joint infection where a negative examination essentially excludes infection.

GALLIUM SCINTIGRAPHY

Gallium is an old and poorly understood tracer, which accumulates in areas of active inflammation and infection. Uptake likely reflects a combination of increased blood flow, membrane permeability, lactoferrin binding, and bacterial uptake.[9] Gallium imaging is performed 18 to 72 hours after tracer injection, making it a less desirable examination. Gallium imaging for infection is essentially limited to spinal infections, where it is often combined with a bone scan. This imaging can be performed when MRI is contraindicated or has equivocal results. The result is considered positive when uptake is greater on gallium than on bone scan.

WHITE BLOOD CELL IMAGING

In vitro–labeled leukocyte imaging can be performed with indium-111 (^{111}In) or ^{99m}Tc. A total white count of at least 2000/μL is needed to obtain satisfactory images.[10] ^{111}In images are acquired 18 to 30 hours after administration, whereas ^{99m}Tc is performed at 4 to 6 hours and repeated at 18 to 30 hours. Leukocytes accumulate in active bone marrow; therefore, its use for detection of spine infection is limited. Variable bone marrow uptake also affects evaluation for periprosthetic joint infection (PJI) when WBC scan is performed alone. This is overcome with the combined or sequential bone marrow imaging with ^{99m}Tc sulfur colloid. Discordant results with uptake on WBC scan and no uptake on bone marrow scan are considered positive for infection.[11]

FLUORINE-18-fluorodeoxyglucose–PET

Fluorine-18-fluorodeoxyglucose (FDG) is taken up into cells via glucose transporters but not metabolized. The degree of uptake is related to the cellular metabolic rate and number of glucose transporters, both of which are high in inflammatory cells. FDG-PET is faster than other nuclear medicine examinations with the examination performed 30 to 60 minutes after tracer injection. Glucose uptake within normal marrow is low; therefore, infection involving the bone is readily seen. The main advantage for FDG-PET seems to be in distinguishing degenerative disc disease from vertebral osteomyelitis and evaluating chronic osteomyelitis. Additionally, because PET is a quantitative imaging method it can be used in treatment monitoring.[12]

MRI

The ability of MRI to evaluate both bone and the adjacent soft tissues make MRI the test of choice in most musculoskeletal infections. Edema is easily identified on fluid-sensitive sequences, which include T2-weighted images (T2WI) and short-tau inversion recovery (STIR). MRI can exclude osteomyelitis with a 100% negative predictive value if the bone marrow is normal on all pulse sequences.[13] MRI can detect acute osteomyelitis as early as 1 to 2 days after onset. Intravenous gadolinium contrast is useful for identifying soft tissue abscesses and sinus tracts, distinguishing synovial thickening from fluid and evaluating spine infections. Gadolinium can show a thick enhancing disc space and help differentiate a paraspinal or epidural phlegmon from an abscess.

SOFT TISSUE INFECTIONS
Cellulitis

Cellulitis is a superficial soft tissue infection involving the skin and subcutaneous tissues. Cellulitis is clinically characterized by soft tissue swelling, erythema, and warmth.[14] Although typically a clinical diagnosis, imaging can help identify extent of disease and exclude more serious conditions such as abscess, myositis, and necrotizing fasciitis. Radiographs are nonspecific and typically show soft tissue swelling with stranding of the subcutaneous fat. Nonetheless, they should be performed first, as they can exclude an underlying foreign body or other unexpected pathologic condition. When there is clinical concern for a more serious infection, MRI is the test of choice because of its excellent soft tissue contrast and ability to identify fluid and edema. On MRI, cellulitis presents as focal or diffuse areas of low signal intensity on T1-weighted images (T1WI) and corresponding high signal intensity on fluid sensitive T2WI within the subcutaneous fat.[2,3] The overlying skin is typically thickened. Enhancement after intravenous gadolinium helps differentiate cellulitis from aseptic edema, such as is seen in congestive heart failure and lymphatic obstruction[2] (**Fig. 1**). CT, which is more readily available and has a shorter imaging time, can be performed as an alternative to MRI. CT shows skin thickening with increased attenuation and enhancement of the subcutaneous fat.[1] Ultrasound scan has a limited role when evaluating soft tissue infection and may underestimate the extent of disease.[15,16] It can demonstrate skin thickening, subcutaneous edema, fluid tracking along the interlobular septa, and hyperemia.[15] Ultrasound scan is typically ordered to exclude deep vein thrombosis or soft tissue abscess.

Necrotizing Fasciitis

Necrotizing fasciitis is a life-threatening soft tissue infection characterized by widespread fascial necrosis. Infections can be either monomicrobial, classically caused by group A *Streptococcus*, or polymicrobial, with mixed aerobic and anaerobic flora. The immunocompromised typically have polymicrobial infections involving the trunk,

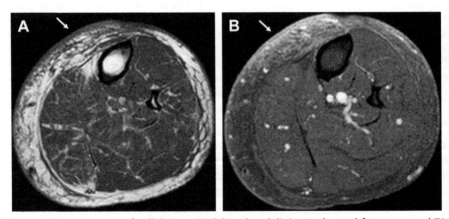

Fig. 1. MRI appearance of cellulitis on T1 (*A*) and gadolinium-enhanced fat-suppressed T1 (*B*) demonstrating skin thickening with underlying subcutaneous edema and enhancement post contrast (*arrows*).

whereas the immunocompetent have monomicrobial infections involving the extremities.[17,18] Clinical presentation includes redness, pain, and swelling, which can be difficult to distinguish from other non-necrotizing soft tissue infections like cellulitis and myositis.[19] Rapid progression, pain disproportionate to degree of swelling and sepsis suggest the diagnosis and may prompt aggressive surgical treatment. Imaging plays a role in equivocal cases and can help delineate the anatomic extent of disease. The presence of soft tissue gas on radiographs is highly specific, but often not present (**Fig. 2**). MRI is the most sensitive examination in identifying soft tissue infections including necrotizing fasciitis. The hallmark of necrotizing fasciitis on MRI is edema of the deep fascia including the intermuscular fascia on T2WI and STIR[20,21] (**Fig. 3**). Kim and colleagues[20] found deep fascial thickening greater than 3 mm in 86% of necrotizing fasciitis cases. There is variable enhancement after contrast injection with the mixed pattern being the most common, showing enhancing and nonenhancing portions of the deep fascia.[19,20] Gas in the deep fascial planes is inconsistently seen and would result in signal voids, best seen on gradient echo sequences.[14] CT is often performed in this rapidly spreading, life-threatening condition, because it is more readily available and faster than MRI. CT delineates soft tissue gas better than MRI. It can identify fascial thickening and fluid collections in the deep fascial compartments with variable contrast enhancement.[22]

Pyomyositis/Abscess

Pyomyositis is a pyogenic infection of the skeletal muscle that leads to muscle swelling and eventually abscess formation. An abscess can occur in the superficial or deep soft tissues and reflects a collection of inflammatory cells, bacteria, and necrotic debris contained by hypervascular connective tissue. Superficial abscesses are often secondary to direct inoculation by a puncture injury, whereas intramuscular abscesses or often secondary to hematogenous dissemination. In both instances, the most frequent organism is *Staphylococcus aureus*.[4] Pyogenic muscle infection is typically confined to a single muscle, in contrast to diabetic muscle infarction, which is

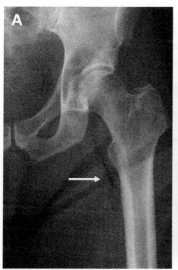
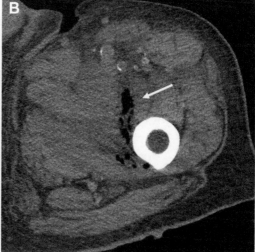

Fig. 2. A 63-year-old man with polymicrobial necrotizing fasciitis. Visible soft tissue gas (*arrows*) on anteroposterior view radiograph (*A*) left hip and CT (*B*).

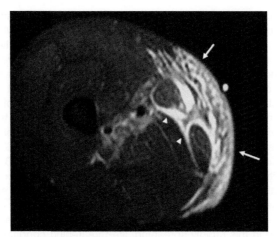

Fig. 3. A 40-year-old man with group A Streptococcus necrotizing fasciitis. MRI axial STIR image shows skin thickening and subcutaneous edema (*arrows*) and fluid extending deep into the intermuscular fascia (*arrowheads*).

often bilateral.[2] However, in up to 40% of patients, multiple muscles can be seeded hematogenously.[23]

Radiographs are typically normal; however, when large enough, an abscess can appear masslike on radiographs. Soft tissue gas or an air-fluid level can sometimes be seen and suggests an abscess.[14,24] Rarely, a periosteal reaction or joint effusion can be seen when the abscess is located adjacent to the bone or joint.[24] MRI is superb at evaluating deep soft tissue infections including pyomyositis. MRI shows muscle enlargement with heterogeneously low signal on T1WI and edema manifested by increased signal on fluid-sensitive sequences. An intramuscular phlegmon will appear as poorly marginated increased T2 signal and heterogeneous enhancement. If an abscess forms, it will appear as a peripherally enhancing superficial or intramuscular fluid collection with intermediate-to-low signal on T1WI and high signal on T2WI and STIR[2] (**Fig. 4**). There is peripheral enhancement on the postcontrast images of the thick irregular wall. CT findings include enlargement of the muscle or muscles along with

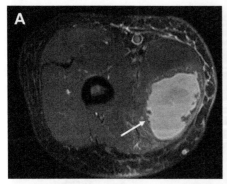
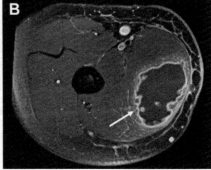

Fig. 4. Pyomyositis with an intramuscular abscess (*arrows*) characterized by well-circumscribed high signal fluid collection on fat-suppressed T2 (*A*) and peripheral enhancement on the gadolinium-enhanced fat-suppressed T1 (*B*).

effacement of the intramuscular and intermuscular fat planes. Postcontrast CT will show enhancement of the affected muscle with or without associated fluid collections.[25] A fluid collection with a thick enhancing wall and presence of soft tissue gas within the collection is diagnostic of an abscess.[1] Ultrasound scan is an excellent modality for identifying soft tissue abscesses, especially if superficial (**Fig. 5**). Ultrasound scan will show a well-delineated fluid collection with a hyperechoic wall. Both ultrasound scan and CT have the added advantage of providing image guidance for aspiration or drainage when necessary.

SEPTIC ARTHRITIS, BURSITIS, AND TENOSYNOVITIS
Septic Arthritis

Septic arthritis is most often secondary to hematogenous seeding; direct inoculation from trauma or surgery is less common. Greater than 50% of cases are secondary to *S aureus*.[26] Clinically, patients present with sudden-onset pain with a warm, swollen joint, decreased range of motion, and inability to bear weight. Fever and chills are not always present. The knee is the most commonly involved joint followed by the hip, ankle, wrist, shoulder, and elbow.[27] Rapid diagnosis and treatment are essential, as delay may result in irreversible cartilage damage.

Radiographs should always be performed and may detect a joint effusion. With disease progression, periarticular osteopenia, joint space narrowing secondary to cartilage loss, and marginal erosions develop (**Fig. 6**). Joint effusions can be identified on radiographs in the knees, elbows, and ankles. Radiographs cannot reliably identify joint effusions in the hips, shoulders, wrists, or small joints. Furthermore, evaluation of the sternoclavicular and sacroiliac joints is severely limited on radiographs because of overlying soft tissues. In these cases, further evaluation with MRI or CT is necessary. The presence of a joint effusion should prompt an arthrocentesis, whether at the bedside or under image guidance. Image guidance is typically performed under fluoroscopy or ultrasound scan. Ultrasound scan is highly sensitive for fluid and can show a joint effusion with associated hyperemia and help guide aspiration.[16] It is the preferred method of hip aspiration in pediatrics.[28] Of note, ultrasound scan is user dependent, and the modality used for guidance should be chosen by the physician performing the aspiration. CT can be used for aspiration of the sternoclavicular and sacroiliac joints. The aspirated fluid should routinely be sent for cell count and

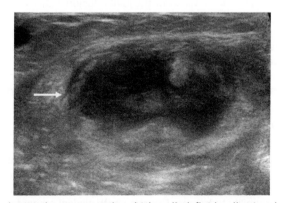

Fig. 5. Ultrasound scan shows a complex thick-walled fluid collection (*arrow*) consistent with the intramuscular abscess in **Fig. 4**. Abscess was aspirated under ultrasound guidance and cultures grew *Streptococcus viridans*.

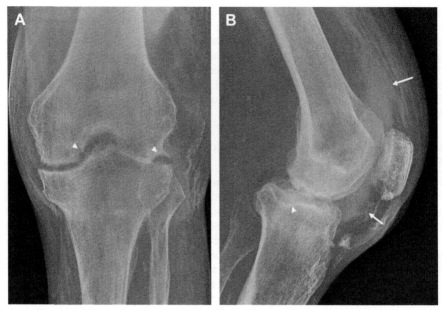

Fig. 6. Septic arthritis in a 59-year-old man with methicillin-sensitive *S aureus*. Anteroposterior (*A*) and lateral (*B*) radiographs show advanced findings of septic arthritis including a joint effusion (*arrows*), erosions (*arrowheads*), and periarticular osteopenia.

differential, crystals, Gram stain, and aerobic and anaerobic cultures. In the appropriate clinical setting, mycobacterial and fungal cultures should also be sent for evaluation. As much fluid as possible should be aspirated, as this helps decompress the joint and alleviate symptoms.[27] If no fluid is obtained, a lavage should be performed irrigating the joint with nonbacteriostatic solution in attempt to obtain a sample. The lavaged sample can be sent for cultures.

MRI is not routinely used in the workup of septic arthritis despite a 100% sensitivity and ability to show changes as early as 24 hours after onset of symptoms.[26,29] It lacks specificity, and findings are indistinguishable from inflammatory arthritis and immune-mediated/viral synovitis.[30] MRI will show the joint effusion with low signal intensity on T1WI and high signal intensity on T2WI. Thickened enhancing synovium is present on postcontrast images in 98% of cases.[26] Subchondral marrow changes and perisynovial soft tissue edema favor infection but are not always present[30] (**Fig. 7**). CT is rarely used for suspected septic arthritis, with the exception of the sternoclavicular and sacroiliac joints where it can show erosions or sclerosis. Surrounding soft tissue edema, joint effusions, or adjacent fluid collections can also be seen.

Septic Bursitis and Tenosynovitis

Septic bursitis and tenosynovitis generally occur in the setting of recent trauma or needle puncture. As with septic arthritis, *S aureus* is the most common infectious agent.[31] Fungal and mycobacterial infections are less commonly encountered. The olecranon and prepatellar bursae are most frequently involved secondary to their superficial location and susceptibility to trauma. Because both clinical presentation and imaging appearance may be indistinguishable from inflammatory aseptic bursitis and tenosynovitis, aspiration is often required.

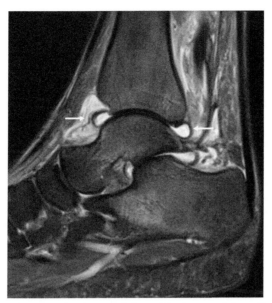

Fig. 7. Fat-suppressed T2-weighted MRI of the ankle shows a joint effusion (*arrows*) surrounded by soft tissue edema and mild marrow edema. Aspiration confirmed septic arthritis and grew *Candida parapsilosis.*

Radiographs are nonspecific but typically show soft tissue swelling and obliteration of the adjacent fat planes (**Fig. 8**). Ultrasound scan can show the distended bursa or tendon sheath with surrounding hyperemia and can help guide aspiration. MRI will show the distended bursa or tendon sheath with low signal intensity on T1WI and

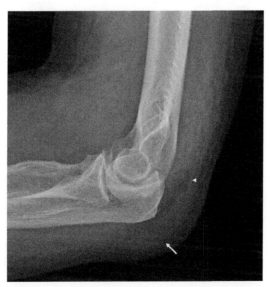

Fig. 8. Lateral radiograph of the elbow shows a distended olecranon bursa (*arrow*) with associated soft tissue gas in the bursa (*arrowhead*) diagnostic of septic bursitis. Intraoperative cultures grew methicillin-sensitive *S aureus.*

high signal intensity on T2WI. Low signal intensity rice bodies can be seen within the fluid, which are found in both rheumatoid arthritis and mycobacterial infections[4] (**Fig. 9**). Thickened enhancing synovium is present on postcontrast images, and air bubbles can be seen as signal voids within the affected bursa or tendon sheath. CT can show the distended bursa or tendon sheath with variable enhancement and is the most sensitive in detecting small amounts of gas. CT can also show inflammatory changes in the surrounding soft tissue and potential ulcerations or sinus tracts.

PERIPROSTHETIC JOINT INFECTIONS

Joint arthroplasty is a tremendously successful operation that has relieved pain and improved the quality of life for millions. With an aging population and growing trend of joint replacement in younger patients, the number of joint arthroplasties performed annually is increasing and is currently more than 1 million per year within the United States.[32] PJI remains a major cause of failure, occurring in 0.3% to 2% of arthroplasties and up to 20% of revisions.[33] Diagnosis of PJI remains a clinical challenge with devastating consequences if missed. Significance of PJI is underscored by the fact that both the American Academy of Orthopedic Surgeons and the Musculoskeletal Infection Society produced guidelines on the diagnosis of PJI in 2011 and 2013,

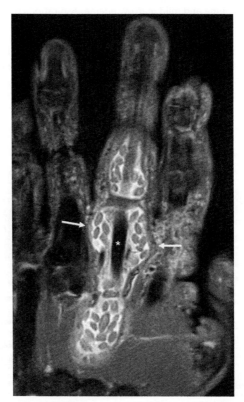

Fig. 9. Septic tenosynovitis of the third flexor digitorum tendon (*asterisk*) in a 64-year-old man with history of puncture wound. Coronal STIR MRI shows a distended fluid-filled tendon sheath and multiple rice bodies (*arrows*). Cultures grew *Mycobacterium marinum*.

respectively.[34,35] Guidelines recommend radiographs and joint aspiration when evaluating for PJI; however, other imaging modalities are not routinely endorsed.

Radiographs are the initial examination performed when evaluating all orthopedic hardware, including joint replacements. Although of low sensitivity and specificity, radiographs can assess the type of implant and hardware used and potentially rule out other causes of joint pain. Common radiographic findings of PJI include periprosthetic lucency of greater than 2 mm at the bone-cement or bone-metal interface indicative of osteolysis[36] (Fig. 10). This finding, however, can be seen with both septic and aseptic loosening. More rapid progression of the periprosthetic lucency, cement fractures, and periosteal reaction support diagnosis of infection.[37]

Radiographs are followed by joint aspiration, either at bedside or under image guidance. Fluoroscopy has the advantage of using contrast injection to delineate potential sinus tracts or extravasation in cases of joint dehiscence (Fig. 11). Aspirated fluid should be sent for Gram stain, aerobic/anaerobic cultures, and cell count with differential. Cultures can include mycobacterial and fungal cultures in at-risk patients or when clinical suspicion dictates. Additional tests of the synovial fluid such as leukocyte esterase, synovial C-reactive protein, and α-defensin may be performed and improve sensitivity or specificity for PJI.[38–40]

CT and MRI are not part of the routine diagnostic evaluation secondary to artifact from the implanted hardware. However, because radiographs are limited when

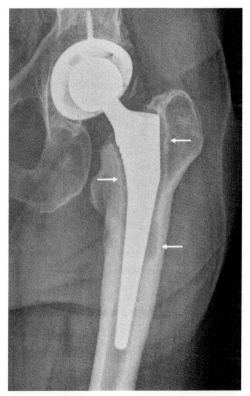

Fig. 10. Anteroposterior radiograph of the left total hip arthroplasty with cortical thickening around femoral stem and periprosthetic lucency greater than 2 mm (*arrows*) consistent with loosening. Joint aspiration grew *Propionibacterium acnes*.

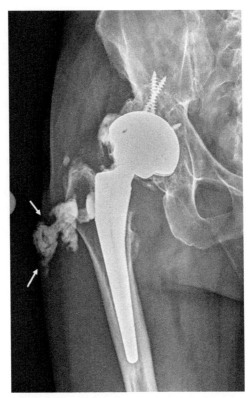

Fig. 11. Anteroposterior radiograph of right total hip arthroplasty after joint aspiration and contrast injection. Injected contrast opacifies the sinus tract (*arrows*), which extends from the hip to the draining wound along the lateral aspect of the thigh.

evaluating the surrounding soft tissues, CT and MRI may be used in complex cases with suspected soft tissue abscesses. Cyteval and colleagues[41] evaluated painful hip prostheses with CT and found that joint distention and periprosthetic fluid collections were accurate for the detection of PJI. Periostitis, when present, was found to be 100% specific, but with a sensitivity of only 16%.[41] With continued advancement in metal artifact reduction techniques and improved image quality, CT and MRI will likely develop into substantial tools in PJI diagnosis in the future.[42]

Although radionuclide imaging is not routinely recommended, it can be used successfully in equivocal cases. ^{99m}Tc 3-phase bone scan can be used as a screening tool because of its high sensitivity. If negative, an infection is considered unlikely, and aseptic etiology for pain should be considered.[11] A positive result is followed by combined or sequential WBC/bone marrow scan. The WBC portion is typically performed with ^{111}In and the bone marrow scintigraphy with ^{99m}Tc sulfur colloid. This combined or sequential WBC/bone marrow scan accounts for the potential uptake of WBC in marrow. Results are positive when there is abnormal uptake on the WBC scan and no uptake of tracer in the same area on the bone marrow scan. Accuracy also increases with the use of SPECT or SPECT-CT, which allows for more precise localization of abnormal uptake.[43] Trevail and colleagues[11] found an accuracy of 97.7% and specificity of 99.5% with this radionuclide imaging algorithm.

OSTEOMYELITIS
Acute Osteomyelitis

Osteomyelitis is a significant form of infection involving the bone or bone marrow in both children and adults that can progress to osteonecrosis, bone destruction, and septic arthritis.[44] The presentation, mode of transmission, and imaging appearance in children and adults differ significantly. This article focuses primarily on adult osteomyelitis with only a few references and key points devoted to pediatric osteomyelitis. Pediatric cases of osteomyelitis are usually secondary to hematogenous spread, bacteremia, in which the bacteria are deposited in the medullary cavity of the long bones. Reactive bone and hypervascular tissue may form around the intramedullary focus of infection developing into an intraosseous abscess, known as a *Brodie abscess*[44] (**Fig. 12**). The bony cortex can eventually rupture, leading to a cortical defect called a *cloaca* and giving rise to a subperiosteal abscess. Subperiosteal abscesses occur more frequently in children, as the cortical bone is thinner and the periosteum is still loosely attached to bone[28,45] (**Fig. 13**). Hematogenous osteomyelitis in adults typically involves the spine and develops into spondylodiskitis, which is discussed separately. In the appendicular skeleton, however, osteomyelitis is caused by contiguous spread from ulcerated skin either owing to vascular insufficiency, neuropathy, or

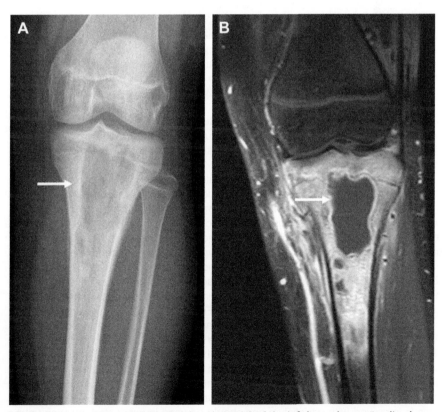

Fig. 12. Anteroposterior radiograph (*A*) and MRI (*B*) of the left knee show a Brodie abscess (*arrows*), which appears as a focal lucency on radiographs and peripherally enhances on the postcontrast fat-suppressed T1WI. There is significant enhancement of the surrounding tibia common in infection.

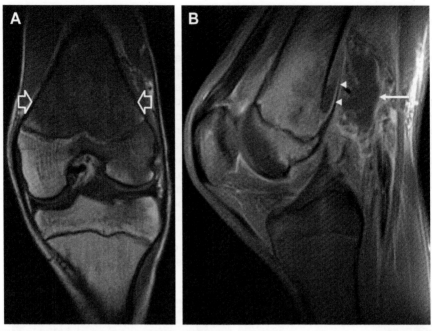

Fig. 13. A 15-year-old with methicillin-sensitive *S aureus* osteomyelitis. T1-weighted (*A*) and postcontrast fat-suppressed T1-weighted (*B*) MRIs show osteomyelitis of the distal femur characterized by confluent low T1 signal (*open arrows*), a subperiosteal abscess (*arrowheads*), and an adjacent soft tissue abscess (*arrow*).

decubiti. Direct inoculation from open fractures, metallic implants, and puncture wounds can be seen in both children and adults and can lead to chronic osteomyelitis.[46] Regardless of age or mode of transmission, *S aureus* is the causative organism in up to 80% of cases.[44]

As previously mentioned, radiographs should be the first imaging examination performed in suspected musculoskeletal infections, including osteomyelitis. Approximately 80% to 95% of radiographs are normal at onset, and up to 90% become positive by 28 days.[45,47] Radiographs can show focal osteopenia, periostitis, permeative bone destruction, or a well circumscribed lucency in the setting of a Brodie abscess. In the setting of contiguous spread, typically seen in pedal osteomyelitis, the earliest radiographic finding is cortical indistinctness (**Fig. 14**). MRI is the most sensitive (82%–100%) and specific (75%–96%) imaging modality for osteomyelitis.[48] Osteomyelitis will appear as an ill-defined low signal marrow replacing process on T1 and corresponding high signal on T2 and STIR (**Fig. 15**). The use of fat suppression increases the conspicuity of pathologic edema associated with osteomyelitis. However, this is not specific and can be seen with bone contusion, fracture, infarct, and tumor. Normal marrow signal on STIR has an almost 100% negative predictive value for osteomyelitis. The use of intravenous gadolinium is still debated and often not used in adults with renal insufficiency, which is common in the patients at risk for osteomyelitis. Although not essential for diagnosing osteomyelitis, the evaluation of the soft tissues is improved with gadolinium and should be used in suspected infection unless contraindicated.[49] Gadolinium-enhanced MRI can differentiate a peripherally enhancing abscess from a heterogeneously enhancing phlegmon and detect a sinus tract with peripheral enhancement.[50]

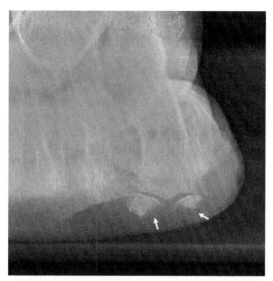

Fig. 14. Radiograph of the hallux sesamoids shows erosions of the sesamoids with loss of the overlying cortex (*arrows*) consistent with osteomyelitis.

Despite superior spatial resolution and ability to identify bony erosions better than MRI, CT is not commonly used for acute osteomyelitis because of poor soft tissue contrast and resulting inability to identify marrow edema and diagnose early osteomyelitis. CT is therefore reserved for cases of chronic osteomyelitis or when MRI is unavailable or contraindicated.

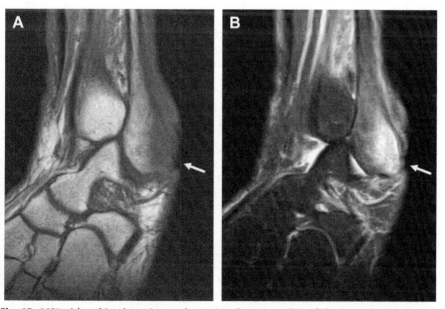

Fig. 15. MRI with a skin ulceration and associated osteomyelitis of the lateral malleolus (*arrows*) characterized by decreased signal on T1WI (*A*) and high signal on the fluid sensitive STIR (*B*).

Ultrasound scan is of limited value in osteomyelitis, as it cannot assess bone. However, in cases of pediatric osteomyelitis, ultrasound scan can identify subperiosteal collections and be used for image-guided aspiration of those collections.[16]

Triple phase bone scan with ^{99m}Tc-methyl diphosphonate has a high sensitivity for detecting osteomyelitis in nonviolated bone, even in early stages of infection. However, specificity is low if the bone has been violated as in trauma or previous surgery, and in these instances, a combined WBC/bone marrow scan is a better test[11] (**Fig. 16**). The combined scan is preferred over the WBC scan alone because it accounts for the variable uptake of white blood cells in normal marrow. The bone marrow scan maps the physiologic uptake of bone marrow, and discordant results with uptake on the WBC scan and no uptake on bone marrow scan indicate infection.

Chronic Osteomyelitis

Chronic osteomyelitis is typically posttraumatic and occurs in 2% to 16% of open fractures and 0.5% to 2% of orthopedic device-related infections.[5] The tibia is the most common site involved. The combination of devitalized bone, hardware, and hematoma is an ideal site for bacterial growth. Radiographs show chronic bone remodeling with cortical thickening, sclerosis, and irregularity. A sequestrum is the most reliable finding for active infection in chronic osteomyelitis.[5] Serial radiographs may be able to detect an interval change with new periosteal reaction or osteolysis to suggest active infection; however, sensitivity and specificity remain low at 14% and 70%, respectively.[51] CT is the best imaging modality for identifying sequestra, involucre, and cloacae in chronic osteomyelitis and should be performed before any planned surgery.[52] The administration of intravenous contrast can help delineate soft tissue sinus tracts or associated abscesses. CT may also help guide a biopsy or aspiration. If a biopsy is planned, it should be performed before the administration of antibiotics or after holding antibiotics for at least 48 hours.[53] MRI can also be used to evaluate chronic osteomyelitis for reactivation or persistent infection, although the specificity (60%) is decreased compared with acute osteomyelitis.[54] Reparative fibrovascular tissue shows similar signal intensity and enhancement characteristics, as active infection and can persist for up to 12 months.[5] Secondary signs of infection must be used to increase diagnostic accuracy and include cutaneous ulcers, sinus tracts, abscess formation, and cortical disruption[55] (**Fig. 17**). Gadolinium-enhanced MRI is especially useful in chronic osteomyelitis, as areas of active inflammation will enhance.[56] Furthermore, sequestra are surrounded by hypervascular granulation tissue with peripheral enhancement. An involucrum appears as a thickened shell of bone around the sequestra with or without marrow edema.[44] The radionuclide test of choice in chronic osteomyelitis is FDG-PET with a reported sensitivity and specificity up to 100% and 95%, respectively.[57] Furthermore, FDG-PET can distinguish between aseptic nonunion of fracture and osteomyelitis.[57] The initial disadvantage of poor anatomic localization has been resolved with the increased use and availability of PET-CT.

SPINE INFECTIONS
Spondylodiscitis

Spondylodiscitis or vertebral osteomyelitis is the most frequent spine infection typically involving 2 adjacent vertebral bodies and the intervening disc. The incidence of spondylodiscitis is increasing secondary to an aging population, inherent comorbidities, and increased use of advanced imaging such as MRI.[58,59] Most cases arise from hematogenous seeding of the axial skeleton from remote infected foci.[60] Less frequently it can arise from contiguous spread from adjacent soft tissues or direct

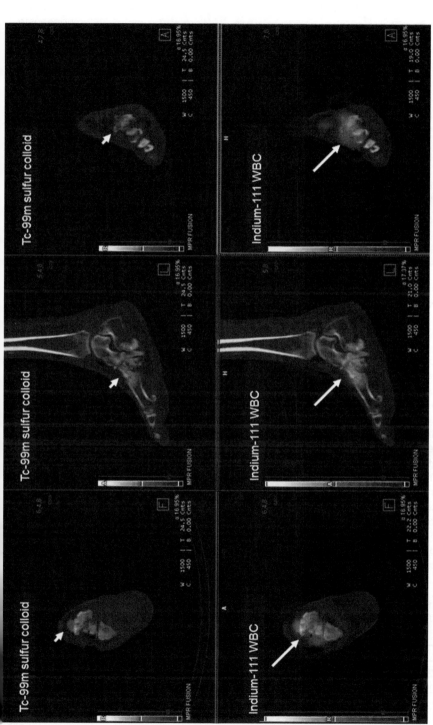

Fig. 16. Combined ^{99m}Tc sulfur colloid (*top*) and ^{111}In WBC (*bottom*) scan for suspected infected neuropathic joint. Imaging performed with combined SPECT-CT for improved localization. Minimal uptake (*short arrows*) on the sulfur colloid bone marrow scan and significant uptake (*long arrows*) on the ^{111}In WBC scan consistent with infection. (*Courtesy of* Dr Donald Neumann, Cleveland Clinic, Cleveland, OH.)

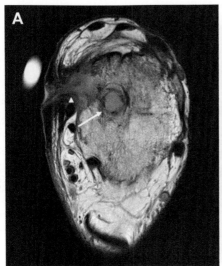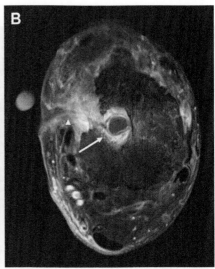

Fig. 17. Chronic methicillin-resistant *S aureus* osteomyelitis in a 42-year-old man with history of remote trauma and surgery. T1-weighted (*A*) and postcontrast fat-suppressed T1-weighted (*B*) MRI images show an intraosseous abscess (*arrows*) with an associated cloaca and sinus tract (*arrowhead*). There is visible enhancement of the fibrovascular tissue surrounding the abscess and sinus tract.

inoculation during spinal instrumentation.[61] The infection starts along the anterior aspect of the vertebral body adjacent to the anterior longitudinal ligament, quickly spreading across the intervening disc space into the adjacent vertebral body. Spread into the adjoining soft tissues accounts for the development of epidural, paravertebral muscle and psoas muscle abscesses.[62] Clinical presentation includes back pain and restricted mobility. Inflammatory markers like erythrocyte sedimentation rate and C-reactive protein are often elevated; however, fever is present in less than half of patients.[63,64] Average delay in diagnosis is 1 to 3 months.[65]

The first examination performed should be radiographs, although they likely will be normal at disease onset. Findings are only visible after several weeks and include decreased bone density, disc space narrowing with endplate destruction, and ultimately subluxation and instability. MRI is the best imaging modality with a sensitivity and specificity of greater than 90%.[61,66] MRI findings of spondylodiscitis are listed in **Table 1** and include disc space narrowing with increased signal on T2WI and enhancement after contrast.

Table 1
MRI features of spondylodiscitis

MRI Findings of Spondylodiscitis			
	T1	**T2**	**T1 + Gd**
Disc space	Dark	Bright[a]	Enhance[a]
Endplates	Dark	Bright	Enhance
Paraspinal	Intermediate	Bright[a]	Enhance
Epidural	Dark	Bright	Enhance

[a] The most sensitive features.

The endplates show low T1 signal, high T2 signal and enhancement postcontrast (**Fig. 18**). Endplate destruction may be present, although this is better seen on CT. Paraspinal soft tissue inflammation is seen as high T2 signal and enhancement, which helps differentiate spondylodiscitis from degenerative disc disease.[67] Epidural enhancement with or without an epidural phlegmon or abscess is commonly seen with spondylodiscitis (**Fig. 19**). Gadolinium should always be used when possible and is essential in differentiating between a phlegmon and a formed epidural or paraspinal abscess.[68] Disc space enhancement is also a highly specific sign for infection and not commonly seen with degenerative change.[61] Additionally, end-plate enhancement can be one of the earliest signs of acute spondylodiscitis.[69]

There is significant overlap between MRI findings in pyogenic and tuberculous spondylodiscitis. Most cases are indistinguishable. Differentiation should be based on clinical history, microbiology, and pathology when available. Nevertheless, there are imaging features that can suggest tuberculous spondylodiscitis. The most specific findings are a well-defined paraspinal abnormality and thin-walled abscess, so-called cold abscess[70] (**Fig. 20**). Additional findings suggesting tuberculous include subligamentous spread and involvement of the thoracic spine.[70]

In cases in which MRI imaging is contraindicated, contrast-enhanced CT scan, PET scan, or combined gallium/^{99m}Tc bone scan can help establish the diagnosis.[7,71,72] Endplate erosions are better seen with CT than MRI and can be performed in equivocal cases or when evaluating for possible biopsy. Intravenous contrast should be used to help evaluate the soft tissues and increase the conspicuity of any abscesses. The major limitation of CT is its inability to evaluate an epidural abscess.[73] Combined gallium/^{99m}Tc bone scan is positive when the gallium uptake is greater than the uptake on bone scan. There is improved localization when SPECT imaging is performed (**Fig. 21**). FDG-PET-CT is the likely best alternative to MRI but is limited secondary to cost and lack of availability. Both FDG-PET and FDG-PET-CT have a comparable sensitivity and specificity to MRI in identifying spondylodiscitis.[74,75] It can also reliably distinguish degenerative modic endplate changes from spondylodiscitis.[72] FDG-PET-CT can also reliably identify psoas and paraspinal abscesses but is inferior to MRI in identifying epidural collections.[75]

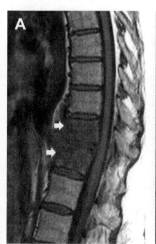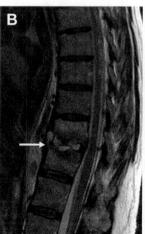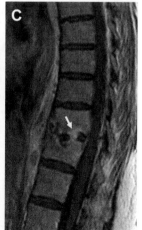

Fig. 18. Typical MRI findings of spondylodiscitis with low signal in the disc space and vertebral bodies (*short arrows*) on T1WI (*A*), high signal within the disc space (*long arrow*) on T2WI (*B*), and enhancement of the disc space (*small arrow*) on postcontrast T1WI (*C*).

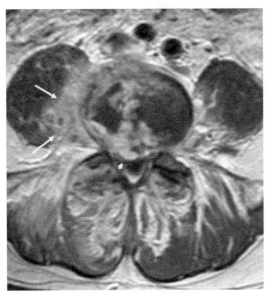

Fig. 19. T1-weighted gadolinium-enhanced MRI in a 38-year-old man with methicillin-resistant *S aureus* spondylodiscitis shows marked paraspinal (*arrows*) and epidural enhancement (*arrowhead*).

SEPTIC FACET JOINT

A septic facet joint is typically the result of hematogenous seeding of a degenerated spinal facet joint and is frequently overlooked and historically underreported in the literature. The reported incidence has increased in more recent studies with septic facet joints representing 4% to 20% of all spine infections.[76,77] Most cases are

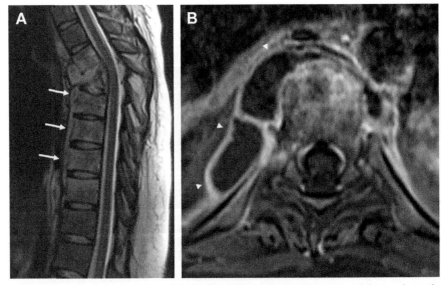

Fig. 20. MRI of tuberculous spondylodiscitis with subligamentous spread (*arrows*) on the T2WI (*A*) and thin walled paraspinal cold abscess (*arrowheads*) on postcontrast T1WI (*B*).

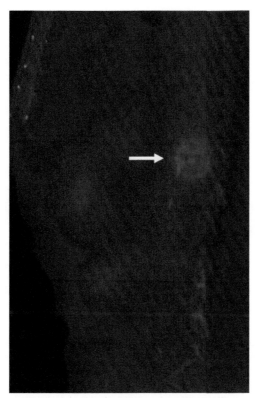

Fig. 21. Gallium-67 SPECT-CT shows focal uptake in the spine at T11-T12 (*arrow*) consistent with spondylodiscitis. (*Courtesy of* Dr Donald Neumann, Cleveland Clinic, Cleveland, OH.)

hematogenous, whereas a small subset is iatrogenic, secondary to local facet injections or instrumentation. Presentation differs from spondylodiscitis with a more acute onset of unilateral back pain with or without associated radicular pain. Unlike spondylodiscitis cases, patients with a septic facet joint are more likely to be febrile (>80%).[76] Furthermore, the causative organism is found in most cases, with the yield of aspirates and tissue cultures of more than 75%. Combined blood culture and aspirate yields causative organism in greater than 90% of cases.[76] Similar to spondylodiscitis, the most frequently isolated organism is *S aureus*.

Radiographs will typically be normal or show degenerative changes of the facet joints. Erosive changes and irregularities at the facet joint are difficult to identify even when present and may not be identified for 6 to 12 weeks.[78,79] MRI is the best examination for evaluating suspected septic facet joints and can establish a diagnosis as early as 5 days after onset of symptoms.[80,81] MRI shows fluid in the facet joint with associated edema of the involved facets and adjacent soft tissues (**Fig. 22**). The edema is most conspicuous on fluid-sensitive sequences, including fat-suppressed T2WI and STIR. Gadolinium is essential for identifying epidural and paraspinal abscesses, which are often associated with the septic facet joint (**Fig. 23**). The frequency of associated epidural abscesses has been reported between 25% and 60% and typically involves the posterior epidural space adjacent to the facet joint.[76,77,82] The paraspinal abscess usually involves the posterior paraspinal musculature. If MRI is

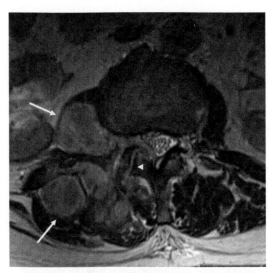

Fig. 22. T2-weighted MRI shows right paraspinal and psoas fluid collections (*arrows*) arising from the right-sided lumbar facet (*arrowhead*). There is posterior epidural thickening abutting the thecal sac without an abscess.

contraindicated or unavailable, CT with contrast can be performed and shows erosive changes in affected facets as well as additional soft tissue inflammatory changes and can delineate the extent of paraspinal or psoas muscle involvement.[83,84] Both positive ^{99m}Tc bone scans and gallium-67 scintigraphy have been reported in affected facets.[82,83,85] The uptake pattern differs from that of spondylodiscitis with the focus of uptake being to one side of midline and more intense on the posterior projection.[82] Similar results would be expected with FDG-PET and localization improved with SPECT.

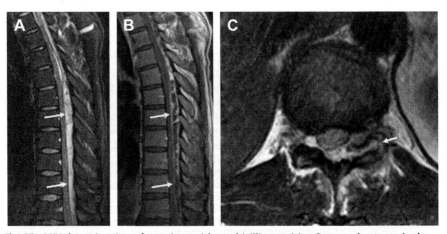

Fig. 23. MRI thoracic spine of a patient with methicillin-sensitive *S aureus* bacteremia shows a large epidural abscess (*arrows*) on the sagittal T2WI (*A*) and peripheral enhancement of the epidural abscess (*arrows*) on the postcontrast T1WI (*B*). The source of the epidural is a septic thoracic facet joint (*small arrow*) seen on the axial T2WI (*C*).

REFERENCES

1. Fayad LM, Carrino JA, Fishman EK. Musculoskeletal infection: role of CT in the emergency department. Radiographics 2007;27(6):1723–36.
2. Yu JS, Habib P. MR imaging of urgent inflammatory and infectious conditions affecting the soft tissues of the musculoskeletal system. Emerg Radiol 2009; 16(4):267–76.
3. Rahmouni A, Chosidow O, Mathieu D, et al. MR imaging in acute infectious cellulitis. Radiology 1994;192(2):493–6.
4. Beltran J. MR imaging of soft-tissue infection. Magn Reson Imaging Clin N Am 1995;3(4):743–51.
5. Kaim AH, Gross T, von Schulthess GK. Imaging of chronic posttraumatic osteomyelitis. Eur Radiol 2002;12(5):1193–202.
6. Riebel TW, Nasir R, Nazarenko O. The value of sonography in the detection of osteomyelitis. Pediatr Radiol 1996;26(4):291–7.
7. Palestro CJ, Torres MA. Radionuclide imaging in orthopedic infections. Semin Nucl Med 1997;27(4):334–45.
8. Schauwecker DS. The scintigraphic diagnosis of osteomyelitis. AJR Am J Roentgenol 1992;158(1):9–18.
9. Palestro CJ. Nuclear medicine and the failed joint replacement: past, present, and future. World J Radiol 2014;6(7):446–58.
10. Palestro CJ, Love C, Miller TT. Infection and musculoskeletal conditions: Imaging of musculoskeletal infections. Best Pract Res Clin Rheumatol 2006;20(6): 1197–218.
11. Trevail C, Ravindranath-Reddy P, Sulkin T, et al. An evaluation of the role of nuclear medicine imaging in the diagnosis of periprosthetic infections of the hip. Clin Radiol 2016;71(3):211–9.
12. Kalicke T, Schmitz A, Risse JH, et al. Fluorine-18 fluorodeoxyglucose PET in infectious bone diseases: results of histologically confirmed cases. Eur J Nucl Med 2000;27(5):524–8.
13. Craig JG, Amin MB, Wu K, et al. Osteomyelitis of the diabetic foot: MR imaging-pathologic correlation. Radiology 1997;203(3):849–55.
14. Turecki MB, Taljanovic MS, Stubbs AY, et al. Imaging of musculoskeletal soft tissue infections. Skeletal Radiol 2010;39(10):957–71.
15. Chau CL, Griffith JF. Musculoskeletal infections: ultrasound appearances. Clin Radiol 2005;60(2):149–59.
16. Cardinal E, Bureau NJ, Aubin B, et al. Role of ultrasound in musculoskeletal infections. Radiol Clin North Am 2001;39(2):191–201.
17. Endorf FW, Supple KG, Gamelli RL. The evolving characteristics and care of necrotizing soft-tissue infections. Burns 2005;31(3):269–73.
18. Sarani B, Strong M, Pascual J, et al. Necrotizing fasciitis: current concepts and review of the literature. J Am Coll Surg 2009;208(2):279–88.
19. Ali SZ, Srinivasan S, Peh WC. MRI in necrotizing fasciitis of the extremities. Br J Radiol 2014;87(1033):20130560.
20. Kim KT, Kim YJ, Won Lee J, et al. Can necrotizing infectious fasciitis be differentiated from nonnecrotizing infectious fasciitis with MR imaging? Radiology 2011; 259(3):816–24.
21. Malghem J, Lecouvet FE, Omoumi P, et al. Necrotizing fasciitis: contribution and limitations of diagnostic imaging. Joint Bone Spine 2013;80(2):146–54.
22. Schmid MR, Kossmann T, Duewell S. Differentiation of necrotizing fasciitis and cellulitis using MR imaging. AJR Am J Roentgenol 1998;170(3):615–20.

23. Bickels J, Ben-Sira L, Kessler A, et al. Primary pyomyositis. J Bone Joint Surg Am 2002;84-A(12):2277–86.
24. Struk DW, Munk PL, Lee MJ, et al. Imaging of soft tissue infections. Radiol Clin North Am 2001;39(2):277–303.
25. Gordon BA, Martinez S, Collins AJ. Pyomyositis: characteristics at CT and MR imaging. Radiology 1995;197(1):279–86.
26. Karchevsky M, Schweitzer ME, Morrison WB, et al. MRI findings of septic arthritis and associated osteomyelitis in adults. AJR Am J Roentgenol 2004;182(1): 119–22.
27. Lin HM, Learch TJ, White EA, et al. Emergency joint aspiration: a guide for radiologists on call. Radiographics 2009;29(4):1139–58.
28. De Boeck H. Osteomyelitis and septic arthritis in children. Acta Orthop Belg 2005;71(5):505–15.
29. Sandrasegaran K, Saifuddin A, Coral A, et al. Magnetic resonance imaging of septic sacroiliitis. Skeletal Radiol 1994;23(4):289–92.
30. Graif M, Schweitzer ME, Deely D, et al. The septic versus nonseptic inflamed joint: MRI characteristics. Skeletal Radiol 1999;28(11):616–20.
31. Small LN, Ross JJ. Suppurative tenosynovitis and septic bursitis. Infect Dis Clin North Am 2005;19(4):991–1005, xi.
32. Hall MJ, DeFrances CJ, Williams SN, et al. National Hospital Discharge Survey: 2007 summary. Natl Health Stat Report 2010;(29):1–20, 24.
33. Nodzo SR, Bauer T, Pottinger PS, et al. Conventional diagnostic challenges in periprosthetic joint infection. J Am Acad Orthop Surg 2015;23(Suppl):S18–25.
34. Della Valle C, Parvizi J, Bauer TW, et al. American Academy of Orthopaedic Surgeons clinical practice guideline on: the diagnosis of periprosthetic joint infections of the hip and knee. J Bone Joint Surg Am 2011;93(14):1355–7.
35. Zmistowski B, Della Valle C, Bauer TW, et al. Diagnosis of periprosthetic joint infection. J Arthroplasty 2014;29(2 Suppl):77–83.
36. Lima AL, Oliveira PR, Carvalho VC, et al. Periprosthetic joint infections. Interdiscip Perspect Infect Dis 2013;2013:542796.
37. Tigges S, Stiles RG, Roberson JR. Appearance of septic hip prostheses on plain radiographs. AJR Am J Roentgenol 1994;163(2):377–80.
38. Aggarwal VK, Tischler E, Ghanem E, et al. Leukocyte esterase from synovial fluid aspirate: a technical note. J Arthroplasty 2013;28(1):193–5.
39. Parvizi J, McKenzie JC, Cashman JP. Diagnosis of periprosthetic joint infection using synovial C-reactive protein. J Arthroplasty 2012;27(8 Suppl):12–6.
40. Deirmengian C, Kardos K, Kilmartin P, et al. The alpha-defensin test for periprosthetic joint infection responds to a wide spectrum of organisms. Clin Orthop Relat Res 2015;473(7):2229–35.
41. Cyteval C, Hamm V, Sarrabere MP, et al. Painful infection at the site of hip prosthesis: CT imaging. Radiology 2002;224(2):477–83.
42. Gupta A, Subhas N, Primak AN, et al. Metal artifact reduction: standard and advanced magnetic resonance and computed tomography techniques. Radiol Clin North Am 2015;53(3):531–47.
43. van der Bruggen W, Bleeker-Rovers CP, Boerman OC, et al. PET and SPECT in osteomyelitis and prosthetic bone and joint infections: a systematic review. Semin Nucl Med 2010;40(1):3–15.
44. Lee YJ, Sadigh S, Mankad K, et al. The imaging of osteomyelitis. Quant Imaging Med Surg 2016;6(2):184–98.
45. Jaramillo D. Infection: musculoskeletal. Pediatr Radiol 2011;41(Suppl 1): S127–34.

46. Calhoun JH, Manring MM. Adult osteomyelitis. Infect Dis Clin North Am 2005; 19(4):765–86.
47. Wheat J. Diagnostic strategies in osteomyelitis. Am J Med 1985;78(6B):218–24.
48. Santiago Restrepo C, Gimenez CR, McCarthy K. Imaging of osteomyelitis and musculoskeletal soft tissue infections: current concepts. Rheum Dis Clin North Am 2003;29(1):89–109.
49. Pugmire BS, Shailam R, Gee MS. Role of MRI in the diagnosis and treatment of osteomyelitis in pediatric patients. World J Radiol 2014;6(8):530–7.
50. Donovan A, Schweitzer ME. Use of MR imaging in diagnosing diabetes-related pedal osteomyelitis. Radiographics 2010;30(3):723–36.
51. Tumeh SS, Aliabadi P, Weissman BN, et al. Disease activity in osteomyelitis: role of radiography. Radiology 1987;165(3):781–4.
52. Ledermann HP, Kaim A, Bongartz G, et al. Pitfalls and limitations of magnetic resonance imaging in chronic posttraumatic osteomyelitis. Eur Radiol 2000; 10(11):1815–23.
53. Mader JT, Cripps MW, Calhoun JH. Adult posttraumatic osteomyelitis of the tibia. Clin Orthop Relat Res 1999;(360):14–21.
54. Kaim A, Ledermann HP, Bongartz G, et al. Chronic post-traumatic osteomyelitis of the lower extremity: comparison of magnetic resonance imaging and combined bone scintigraphy/immunoscintigraphy with radiolabelled monoclonal antigranulocyte antibodies. Skeletal Radiol 2000;29(7):378–86.
55. Morrison WB, Schweitzer ME, Batte WG, et al. Osteomyelitis of the foot: relative importance of primary and secondary MR imaging signs. Radiology 1998; 207(3):625–32.
56. Dangman BC, Hoffer FA, Rand FF, et al. Osteomyelitis in children: gadolinium-enhanced MR imaging. Radiology 1992;182(3):743–7.
57. Guhlmann A, Brecht-Krauss D, Suger G, et al. Fluorine-18-FDG PET and technetium-99m antigranulocyte antibody scintigraphy in chronic osteomyelitis. J Nucl Med 1998;39(12):2145–52.
58. Akiyama T, Chikuda H, Yasunaga H, et al. Incidence and risk factors for mortality of vertebral osteomyelitis: a retrospective analysis using the Japanese diagnosis procedure combination database. BMJ Open 2013;3(3):e002412.
59. Kehrer M, Pedersen C, Jensen TG, et al. Increasing incidence of pyogenic spondylodiscitis: a 14-year population-based study. J Infect 2014;68(4):313–20.
60. Nickerson EK, Sinha R. Vertebral osteomyelitis in adults: an update. Br Med Bull 2016;117(1):121–38.
61. Sans N, Faruch M, Lapegue F, et al. Infections of the spinal column–spondylodiscitis. Diagn Interv Imaging 2012;93(6):520–9.
62. Hadjipavlou AG, Mader JT, Necessary JT, et al. Hematogenous pyogenic spinal infections and their surgical management. Spine (Phila Pa 1976) 2000;25(13): 1668–79.
63. Mrabet D, Mizouni H, Khiari H, et al. Brucellar spondylodiscitis affecting non-contiguous spine levels. BMJ Case Rep 2011;2011.
64. Siemionow K, Steinmetz M, Bell G, et al. Identifying serious causes of back pain: cancer, infection, fracture. Cleve Clin J Med 2008;75(8):557–66.
65. Cottle L, Riordan T. Infectious spondylodiscitis. J Infect 2008;56(6):401–12.
66. Dagirmanjian A, Schils J, McHenry M, et al. MR imaging of vertebral osteomyelitis revisited. AJR Am J Roentgenol 1996;167(6):1539–43.
67. Diehn FE. Imaging of spine infection. Radiol Clin North Am 2012;50(4):777–98.
68. Ledermann HP, Schweitzer ME, Morrison WB, et al. MR imaging findings in spinal infections: rules or myths? Radiology 2003;228(2):506–14.

69. Dunbar JA, Sandoe JA, Rao AS, et al. The MRI appearances of early vertebral osteomyelitis and discitis. Clin Radiol 2010;65(12):974–81.
70. Jung NY, Jee WH, Ha KY, et al. Discrimination of tuberculous spondylitis from pyogenic spondylitis on MRI. AJR Am J Roentgenol 2004;182(6):1405–10.
71. Love C, Patel M, Lonner BS, et al. Diagnosing spinal osteomyelitis: a comparison of bone and Ga-67 scintigraphy and magnetic resonance imaging. Clin Nucl Med 2000;25(12):963–77.
72. Ohtori S, Suzuki M, Koshi T, et al. 18F-fluorodeoxyglucose-PET for patients with suspected spondylitis showing Modic change. Spine (Phila Pa 1976) 2010; 35(26):E1599–603.
73. Prodi E, Grassi R, Iacobellis F, et al. Imaging in Spondylodiskitis. Magn Reson Imaging Clin N Am 2016;24(3):581–600.
74. Prodromou ML, Ziakas PD, Poulou LS, et al. FDG PET is a robust tool for the diagnosis of spondylodiscitis: a meta-analysis of diagnostic data. Clin Nucl Med 2014;39(4):330–5.
75. Smids C, Kouijzer IJ, Vos FJ, et al. A comparison of the diagnostic value of MRI and 18F-FDG-PET/CT in suspected spondylodiscitis. Infection 2017;45(1):41–9.
76. Muffoletto AJ, Ketonen LM, Mader JT, et al. Hematogenous pyogenic facet joint infection. Spine (Phila Pa 1976) 2001;26(14):1570–6.
77. Narvaez J, Nolla JM, Narvaez JA, et al. Spontaneous pyogenic facet joint infection. Semin Arthritis Rheum 2006;35(5):272–83.
78. Halpin DS, Gibson RD. Septic arthritis of a lumbar facet joint. J Bone Joint Surg Br 1987;69(3):457–9.
79. Roberts WA. Pyogenic vertebral osteomyelitis of a lumbar facet joint with associated epidural abscess. A case report with review of the literature. Spine (Phila Pa 1976) 1988;13(8):948–52.
80. Pilleul F, Garcia J. Septic arthritis of the spine facet joint: early positive diagnosis on magnetic resonance imaging. Review of two cases. Joint Bone Spine 2000; 67(3):234–7.
81. Andre V, Pot-Vaucel M, Cozic C, et al. Septic arthritis of the facet joint. Med Mal Infect 2015;45(6):215–21.
82. Ergan M, Macro M, Benhamou CL, et al. Septic arthritis of lumbar facet joints. A review of six cases. Rev Rhum Engl Ed 1997;64(6):386–95.
83. Tay BK, Deckey J, Hu SS. Spinal infections. J Am Acad Orthop Surg 2002;10(3): 188–97.
84. Tali ET, Gultekin S. Spinal infections. Eur Radiol 2005;15(3):599–607.
85. Swayne LC, Dorsky S, Caruana V, et al. Septic arthritis of a lumbar facet joint: detection with bone SPECT imaging. J Nucl Med 1989;30(8):1408–11.

Osteomyelitis

Steven K. Schmitt, MD

KEYWORDS

- Osteomyelitis • Diabetic foot infection • Hematogenous osteomyelitis
- Traumatic osteomyelitis • MRSA

KEY POINTS

- Hematogenous osteomyelitis is the most common presentation in children and is often medically treated, although methicillin-resistant *Staphylococcus aureus* infections may require surgery.
- Staging of osteomyelitis addresses both the extent of the disease and the underlying health of the host, and can help to suggest appropriate management steps.
- Probing to bone has a high correlation with infection in diabetic foot ulcers. Cross-sectional techniques such as MRI can suggest a diagnosis when clinical presentation is less clear.
- Appropriate treatment of diabetic foot infections includes assessment of vascular supply as part of the decision making regarding surgical debridement.
- Established infections in patients with open fractures may present as nonunion and require a combination of medical and surgical treatments.

INTRODUCTION AND HISTORY

Osteomyelitis is an infection of the bone. Several major syndromes are commonly seen, including hematogenous osteomyelitis, vertebral osteomyelitis (discussed elsewhere in this issue), osteomyelitis after trauma, and diabetic foot infection.

Osteomyelitis is an ancient disease, with fossilized evidence of animal infection hundreds of millions of years ago. Discussion of human osteomyelitis dates to the time of Hippocrates (460–370 BC).[1] Acute hematogenous osteomyelitis was called "abscessus in medulla" by Broomfield in 1773.[2] The coining of the term "osteomyelitis" is attributed to Nelaton in 1844.[1] In the preantibiotic era, osteomyelitis management was surgical, with standard of care consisting of debridement, saucerization, and wound packing with secondary healing. With the arrival of penicillin in the 1940s, mortality owing to staphylococcal osteomyelitis improved from around 30% to 10%, with

The author has no relevant disclosures.
Section of Bone and Joint Infections, Department of Infectious Disease, Medicine Institute, Cleveland Clinic, Cleveland Clinic Lerner College of Medicine, 9500 Euclid Avenue, Desk G-21, Cleveland, OH 44195, USA
E-mail address: schmits@ccf.org

Infect Dis Clin N Am 31 (2017) 325–338
http://dx.doi.org/10.1016/j.idc.2017.01.010
0891-5520/17/© 2017 Elsevier Inc. All rights reserved.

id.theclinics.com

the literature evolving to discussion of the relative roles of surgical decompression and antibiotic therapy in the treatment algorithm.

EPIDEMIOLOGY AND CLASSIFICATION

In children, hematogenous osteomyelitis predominates and affects mostly long bones. In younger adults, osteomyelitis is often related to trauma or surgery. In older adults, the most common clinical presentations are contiguous osteomyelitis related to joint arthroplasty (discussed elsewhere in this issue), lower extremity osteomyelitis related to diabetes mellitus and vascular disease, and osteomyelitis related to decubitus ulceration.

There are 2 major classification schemes for osteomyelitis. The first, proposed by Lew and Waldvogel,[3] is based on etiology. In this scheme, osteomyelitis is divided into 3 categories by pathophysiologic mechanism: hematogenous osteomyelitis; contiguous focus osteomyelitis from trauma, surgery, prosthetic material, or soft tissue spread; and vascular insufficiency osteomyelitis often seen in diabetes mellitus.

The second classification scheme, proposed by Cierny and Mader,[4] provides some guidance for management. Osteomyelitis is divided by anatomic stages, and placed in the setting of host health status (**Table 1**). Host health status is defined by local and systemic factors (**Table 2**). Local host factors include edema, circulatory status, tobacco use, and neuropathy, whereas systemic factors include immunocompromising diseases such as neoplasm, organ failure and diabetes, age, and malnutrition. Stage I disease is typically treated with antibiotics, with more advanced stages requiring combined medical and surgical interventions.

PATHOPHYSIOLOGY

Hematogenous osteomyelitis of the long bones usually affects the metaphysis.[5] Slowing of blood flow in vascular loops at the metaphysis near the epiphyseal plates leads to deposition of microbes and establishment of infection. An inflammatory response ensues, leading to increased pressure in the medullary bone. This pressure causes the infection to break through to the cortex and, if unchecked, ultimately through the periosteum. This can lead to decreased blood supply to the periosteum with bone necrosis.

Table 1
Cierny-Mader staging system: anatomic and physiologic types

	Type
Anatomic stage	Anatomic type
1	Medullary
2	Superficial
3	Localized
4	Diffuse
Physiologic host	Physiologic type
A	Normal host
Bs	Systemic compromise
Bl	Local compromise
Bls	Systemic and local compromise
C	Treatment worse than disease

From Cierny G 3rd, Mader JT, Penninck JJ. A clinical staging system for adult osteomyelitis. Clin Orthop Relat Res 2003;(414):7–24; with permission.

Table 2
Cierny–Mader staging system: causes of host compromise

Systemic Compromise (Bs)	Local Compromise (Bl)
Malnutrition	Chronic lymphedema
Renal failure	Venous stasis
Hepatic failure	Major vessel vascular disease
Diabetes mellitus	Small vessel vascular disease
Chronic hypoxia	Arteritis
Immunodeficiency diseases	Peripheral neuropathy
Neoplasm	Tobacco use

From Cierny G 3rd, Mader JT, Penninck JJ. A clinical staging system for adult osteomyelitis. Clin Orthop Relat Res 2003;(414):7–24; with permission.

Pieces of necrotic bone can separate and are called a sequestrum, which can contain pus. New bone can begin to form over the injured periosteum; this is known as an involucrum and may partially surround a sequestrum with ongoing drainage.

Vertebral osteomyelitis most commonly arises from the hematogenous deposition of microbes in the metaphysis of the vertebral bodies. The infection then spreads to the intravertebral disc, which is an avascular structure. Common patterns of infection are often explained by vascular structures, with spread between intramedullary communicating arteries to the metaphyses of a single vertebra and involvement of adjacent vertebral bodies supplied by splitting arteries from a single vertebral artery. Venous drainage via Batson's plexus is felt by some experts to contribute to spondylodiscitis metastasizing from a urinary tract focus.[6]

Diabetes mellitus may lead to compromised microvascular and macrovascular blood supply to the lower extremities. In the setting of the sensory neuropathy that is also common in diabetes mellitus, patients are predisposed to the development of skin ulceration at points of pressure or trauma, with subsequent colonization with skin flora. Poor vasculature contributes to compromised local immunity and skin healing, promoting the spread of infection to the underlying bone.

Patients confined to bed or a wheelchair by paralysis or debility are subject to pressure-related skin ulceration and necrosis, most commonly in the sacral and buttock areas. These ulcerations are colonized frequently by polymicrobial flora emanating from the skin and gastrointestinal tracts, with soft tissue infection spreading to the bones of the pelvis and lower extremities.

Microbial factors also play an important role in osteomyelitis pathogenesis. *Staphylococcus aureus* adhesins, including microbial surface components recognizing adhesive matrix molecules.[7,8] Microbial surface components recognizing adhesive matrix molecules recognize polysaccharides related to fibronectin, fibrinogen, collagen, and heparin, promoting adherence to bone matrix. *S aureus* digested by osteoblasts persist and become more resistant to antimicrobials. Finally, *S aureus* seems to block the inhibition of proteolysis in musculoskeletal structures.

MICROBIOLOGY

Hematogenous osteomyelitis is usually monomicrobial, whereas osteomyelitis related to contiguous spread or inoculation may be monomicrobial or polymicrobial.[9] *S aureus* and coagulase-negative staphylococci are isolated most commonly (**Box 1**) and may originate from distance foci of infection such as skin abscesses or endocarditis, indwelling vascular catheters, or injection drug use. Community-acquired

Box 1
Microbial causes of osteomyelitis in adults

Usual

Staphylococcus aureus

Coagulase-negative Staphylococcus species

Beta-hemolytic streptococci

Viridans streptococci

Enterococci

Aerobic gram-negative bacilli (*Pseudomonas* species, *Enterobacter* species, *Escherichia coli*, others)

Less common

Mycobacterium tuberculosis

Nontuberculous mycobacteria (*Mycobacterium avium intracellulare*, Bacille Calmette Guerin, etc)

Salmonella species

Brucella species

Eikenella corrodens

Candida species

Endemic mycoses (Blastomyces, Coccidioides, Sporothrix)

Cryptococcus species

Aspergillus species

methicillin-resistant *S aureus* (MRSA) has emerged as a pathogen of particular virulence owing to production and tissue release of cytotoxins.[10] Streptococci, enterococci, aerobic gram-negative bacilli, and anaerobes are also commonly encountered. Anaerobic gram-negative bacilli such as peptostreptococci, *Clostridium* species, and *Bacteroides* species may also be found, particularly in polymicrobial infections. *Mycobacterium tuberculosis* may spread to the thoracic spine from a primary infection in the lungs.[11]

A number of pathogens are identified less commonly, but should be considered in the appropriate epidemiologic setting. Nontuberculous mycobacteria are particularly identified in the setting of traumatic injury or immunocompromise. Bacille Calmette-Guerin infection may complicate intravesicular therapy for bladder cancer.[12] *Candida* species may be part of chronic infections after surgery or trauma, in immune compromise, or as a result of hematogenous deposition with indwelling vascular catheters or injection drug use.[13] Dimorphic fungi such as *Blastomyces* species (in the north-central and southern United States) and *Coccidioides* species (in the southwestern United States) may affect the bone in endemic geographic locations. *Cryptococcus* spp and *Aspergillus* spp are found particularly in immunocompromised hosts.[13,14] Bone infections with *Actinomyces* spp[15] and *Sporothrix* spp[13] usually follow traumatic inoculation. *Brucella* spp[16] and *Salmonella* spp[17] are seen in spinal infections. *Salmonella* spp and *S aureus* are common in acute hematogenous osteomyelitis in sickle cell disease.

CLINICAL PRESENTATION

The clinical presentation of osteomyelitis depends on the etiology. Hematogenous osteomyelitis usually presents with subacute or chronic onset of pain at the area of bony involvement. Fever and chills are less common, but can occur with virulent pathogens such as *S aureus*. Soft tissue erythema and swelling and eventually a draining sinus tract may occur, and are particularly prevalent in the setting of trauma/fracture, joint arthroplasty, or nonjoint orthopedic hardware. Infections associated with vascular insufficiency most often present with ulceration, erythema, swelling, and drainage that may progress to visible bone in a subacute to chronic fashion. Infection after an open fracture may present over weeks to months as incomplete wound healing or fracture nonunion. Fever and chills are less common in this setting. Vertebral osteomyelitis typically presents with subacute to chronic pain at the involved site, sometimes with fever. Signs of cord compression and compromise emerge in approximately 25% of patients,[18] with radiating pain from compressed nerve roots corresponding with the involved level, followed by extremity weakness and impaired bowel or bladder function.

DIAGNOSIS

Clinical presentation is a critical part of osteomyelitis diagnosis. In lower extremity osteomyelitis owing to vascular insufficiency, probing to bone is highly suggestive of osteomyelitis. Further confirmation of osteomyelitis usually consists of blood testing, radiologic imaging, and microbiology. In most cases, the erythrocyte sedimentation rate and C-reactive protein are abnormal, though normal with certain indolent pathogens such as *Propionibacterium acnes*. The white blood cell count may be normal or elevated, and anemia with a normocytic, normochromic chronic disease pattern may be present in long-standing infection.

Radiologic imaging is discussed fully in a separate article of this issue. Plain radiographs may have a delay of 10 to 14 days before onset of findings. Cross-sectional imaging such as computed tomography and MRI are sensitive and more specific than plain radiographs. Nuclear imaging studies are sensitive but less specific and often lack anatomic definition necessary to direct surgical management.

Microbiologic diagnosis in acute hematogenous osteomyelitis in children is often made with blood cultures. Because blood cultures are less commonly positive in adults, biopsy is often required, with guidance with computed tomography (CT) imaging or an open procedure.

MANAGEMENT

The treatment of osteomyelitis often requires a combination of medical and surgical management to accomplish a goal of uninfected, pain-free function. Communication and coordination between the surgeon and infectious diseases specialist is essential to creating a unified and effective treatment plan. Because antibiotics penetrate dead or injured bone and infected fluid collections poorly, surgical debridement is a cornerstone of therapy when these are present. In addition to facilitating the penetration of antibiotics into affected bone and soft tissue, debridement also offers other advantages. First, it provides an opportunity to obtain deep tissue culture data to direct antibiotic therapy. Second, because orthopedic hardware creates an avascular surface for microbial colonization, its removal enhances the possibility of microbiological cure. After the removal of infected dead tissue and hardware, nonunion of bone can be addressed where present. Local antibiotic delivery can be initiated by the placement of antibiotic-containing beads or polymethylmethacrylate cement spacers. Finally, dead space can be exposed for flap coverage.

Once surgical control of the affected area has been accomplished, effective antibiotic therapy can be administered (**Table 3**). Vancomycin and a third-generation

Table 3
Pathogen-directed antimicrobial therapy for osteomyelitis in adults[a,b,c]

Organism	Primary Regimens	Alternative Regimens
Staphylococci (*S aureus* or coagulase negative)		
Oxacillin sensitive	Oxacillin or nafcillin 2 g intravenously q4 h Cefazolin 2 g intravenously q8 h	Vancomycin 15 mg/kg q12 h[d] Clindamycin 900 mg intravenously q8 h
Oxacillin resistant	Vancomycin 15 mg/kg q12 h	Clindamycin 900 mg intravenously q8 h Daptomycin 6 mg/kg intravenously daily Linezolid 600 mg intravenously or PO q12 h Levofloxacin 500–750 mg intravenously or PO plus rifampin 300 mg PO BID-TID
Streptococci	Penicillin G 24 million units intravenously continuously or in 6 divided doses Ceftriaxone 2 g intravenously daily Cefazolin 2 g intravenously q8 h	Vancomycin 15 mg/kg q12 h Clindamycin 900 mg intravenously q8 h
Enterococci	Penicillin G 24 million units intravenously continuously or in 6 divided doses	Vancomycin 15 mg/kg q12 h Daptomycin 6 mg/kg intravenously daily Linezolid 600 mg intravenously or PO q12 h
Pseudomonas aeruginosa	Cefepime 2 g intravenously q12 h Ceftazidime 2 g intravenously q8 h	Meropenem 1 g intravenously q8 h Imipenem 500 mg intravenously q6 h Ciprofloxacin 400 mg intravenously or 750 mg PO BID
Enterobacteriaciae (not *P aeruginosa*)	Ceftriaxone 2 g intravenously daily Cefepime 2 g intravenously q12 h Ceftazidime 2 g intravenously q8 h	Ciprofloxacin 400 mg intravenously or 750 mg PO BID Levofloxacin 500–750 mg intravenously or PO daily

Abbreviation: PO, orally.
[a] Typical duration 4 to 6 weeks.
[b] Use antimicrobial susceptibility data to assist with choice.
[c] Based on normal renal function.
[d] Initial dosing; Trough level goal: 15–20 mg/L.

cephalosporin or beta lactam/beta-lactamase inhibitor combination provides broad gram-positive and gram-negative coverage and is the most common empiric regimen pending culture data. When methicillin-susceptible staphylococci are isolated from cultures, penicillinase-resistant penicillins such as oxacillin or nafcillin, or a first-generation cephalosporin such as cefazolin are used commonly. When isolated staphylococci are methicillin resistant, vancomycin is the most commonly used agent. Data regarding the use of newer agents such as daptomycin, linezolid, ceftaroline, dalbavancin, and televancin are emerging.[19] For penicillin-susceptible streptococci or enterococci, penicillin G and ampicillin are used. For gram-negative bacilli that are susceptible, ceftriaxone or ertapenem may be administered once daily for prolonged intravenous therapy. When *Pseudomonas aeruginosa* is isolated, cefepime, ceftazidime, or meropenem are intravenous choices.

There are no good randomized, clinical trials to suggest the use of a single antibiotic or combination of agents for osteomyelitis,[20] and this lack has led to considerable variation in practice. Most experts in the United States recommend 4 to 6 weeks of parenteral antibiotic therapy for osteomyelitis. Once the patient is stable for discharge, treatment can be administered via outpatient parenteral antibiotic therapy with substantial vascular access such as a peripherally inserted central catheter or tunneled Hohn catheter. When gram-negative bacilli are isolated and culture and are fluoroquinolone susceptible, these highly bioavailable agents can be used in high doses as an oral regimen. When infected bone is debrided completely with microbiologic and pathologic suggestion of a clean margin, antibiotic therapy duration can often be reduced. A 2-week course of pathogen-directed parenteral or highly bioavailable oral therapy is adequate to treat residual soft tissue infection, with good clinical follow-up maintained to ensure ongoing improvement.

Hyperbaric oxygen is a controversial adjunctive therapy for osteomyelitis.[21,22] Two mechanisms have been proposed for its action in osteomyelitis. First, increased oxygen tension has direct antimicrobial effect on anaerobic bacteria. Second, it is felt that polymorphonuclear leukocyte killing of organisms is enhanced by increased oxygen tension.

KEY CLINICAL PRESENTATIONS
Vertebral Osteomyelitis

Infections of the spine are a potentially debilitating manifestation of bone infection. The pathophysiology, diagnosis, and management of infections of the disc space, spine, facet joints, and adjacent structures are fully discussed elsewhere in this issue.

Acute Hematogenous Osteomyelitis in Children

Children most often acquire osteomyelitis by the hematogenous route. More than one-half of cases arise before age 5.[23] The long bones are affected most commonly, especially the tibia, femur, and humerus, with the spine accounting for less than 5% of infections.[24] Infections in neonates are related to bacteremia in the setting of indwelling vascular catheters, abnormal urinary anatomy, and skin or soft tissue infection.[25,26] In children older than 3 months of age, sickle cell disease and immunodeficiency related to disease or treatment also may play a role. The most common pathogen (**Table 4**) is S aureus,[27] with community-acquired MRSA playing an increasing role.[10] Streptococcus pneumoniae is prevalent in immunodeficiency states, asplenia, or hyposplenia. In neonates, Escherichia coli and Streptococcus agalactiae (group B) are also common.

Table 4		
Acute hematogenous osteomyelitis in children: microbiology and empiric therapy		
Age	**Pathogen**	**Empiric Regimen**
<3 mo	Staphylococcus aureus Streptococcus agalactiae Escherichia coli	Nafcillin/oxacillin/cefazolin (MSSA predominant areas) or vancomycin/clindamycin (MRSA predominant areas) and cefotaxime
>3 mo	S aureus Streptococcus pneumoniae Streptococcus pyogenes Kingella kingae (to 36 mo)	Nafcillin/oxacillin/cefazolin (MSSA predominant areas) or vancomycin/clindamycin (MRSA predominant areas)

Abbreviations: MRSA, methicillin-resistant Staphylococcus aureus; MSSA, methicillin-susceptible Staphylococcus aureus.

Streptococcus pyogenes infects bones in younger children. There is increased recognition of *Kingella kingae* as a pathogen associated with children aged 6 to 36 months in daycare.[28] *S aureus*, *S pneumoniae*, and *S pyogenes* predominate in older children. Children with indwelling vascular catheters are also prone to infections with health care–associated gram-negative bacilli such as *P aeruginosa*, as well as *Candida albicans* and non-albicans *Candida* species. *Haemophilus influenzae* type B, formerly a common cause of osteomyelitis in children, has nearly disappeared as a pathogen since the introduction of an effective vaccine in 1985.

The pathogenesis of pediatric hematogenous osteomyelitis[29] differs from adults in that the infection is not limited to the metaphyses. Capillary loops form areas of slow flow, with the deposition of organisms from bacteremia, inflammation causing obstruction, and avascular necrosis. Infection spreads through the cortex or growth plate into the joint space. In neonates, a thinner cortex allows rupture into soft tissue. As the cortex thickens with age in older children, there is subperiosteal collection of pus instead of rupture. Diagnosis is radiographic, and microbiology is often established by blood culture but also from surgical cultures when debridement or drainage are performed.

Historically, acute hematogenous osteomyelitis in children has been treated with antimicrobial therapy without surgery. This calculus may be altered for community-acquired MRSA, which may require surgery for control of infection and sepsis. Therapy is usually initiated by the parenteral route (see **Table 4**), with a switch to oral therapy when possible. Duration of therapy is usually 3 weeks. With increased attention to antimicrobial stewardship, there has been a new interest in shorter durations of therapy. Data supporting shorter or longer courses are emerging.[27]

Lower Extremity Osteomyelitis in Patients with Diabetes Mellitus

Patients with diabetes mellitus frequently have complications of ischemic vascular disease and peripheral neuropathy. In this setting, patients are often unaware of pressure phenomena related to footwear fit, with subsequent callus formation and breakdown of normal cutaneous barriers to infection. In addition, patients with neuropathy fail to recognize trauma, increasing the risk of skin breakdown. Once organisms breach the skin barrier, the establishment and spread of infection is promoted by hyperglycemia and decreased vascular supply. Infection spreads to the underlying bone, which may be visible in the ulcer.

Diagnosis is often made by physical examination, with erythema, tenderness, warmth, and swelling, sometimes accompanied by ulceration and purulent drainage. The ability to probe to bone is associated with a high specificity for osteomyelitis, exceeding 90%.[30] Imaging studies, including MRI and nuclear studies, can help to define anatomy and distinguish between infection and the important differential diagnoses of crystalline arthropathy and Charcot arthropathy, although even these advanced modalities can prove troublesome for these differentials.[31] Given the difficulty of healing wounds in poorly vascularized limbs, it is tempting to tailor antimicrobial therapy to the results of swab cultures. This approach has multiple drawbacks. First, there is frequently discordance between wound and deep soft tissue or bone cultures. In addition, swab cultures are inadequate for anaerobic culture. For this reason, the diabetic foot infection guideline of the Infectious Diseases Society of America recommends against the use of swab cultures, especially of undebrided wounds.[32] More accurate microbiologic data are obtained by submission of transcutaneous biopsy or intraoperative specimens for culture. Unfortunately, antibiotic therapy is often initiated before deep cultures are obtained, reducing culture yield.

Together, these factors often lead to inappropriate antibiotic selection, with risk of treatment failure.

Given the polymicrobial nature of diabetic foot infections, broad spectrum coverage is recommended in the empiric situation. Most often used are beta-lactam/beta lactamase inhibitor combinations including ampicillin/sulbactam, piperacillin/tazobactam, and ticarcillin/clavulanate, although a systematic review failed to favor any 1 agent.[21] Because of its favorable pharmacokinetic profile, ertapenem is frequently chosen for longer term parenteral therapy. When the patient has a true beta lactam allergy, a fluoroquinolone may be combined with metronidazole or clindamycin. MRSA coverage (usually vancomycin) should be included in areas with high prevalence or when the patient has a history of MRSA infections. *P aeruginosa* is a consideration when the patient has a history or when the patient has extensive water exposure, including soaking the feet. Antibiotics should be tailored to deep culture results when available. Duration of therapy is often 4 to 6 weeks or longer, but may be shortened to 2 weeks or less with complete debridement of infected tissue and bone. Blood flow to the infected area should always be assessed and interventions undertaken when necessary, given the difficulties of wound healing and antibiotic delivery to infected tissue with impaired vascular supply.

Osteomyelitis After Trauma

Osteomyelitis may develop as a result of contamination of open fractures or open repair of closed fractures.[33] Risk for infection, which occurs in 25% of open fractures, depends on several factors: severity of the fracture, severity of the soft tissue injury, inoculum of bacterial contamination, vascular supply, adequacy of debridement, and administration of prophylactic antibiotics.

Cultures obtained at the time of initial debridement correlate with established pathogens of osteomyelitis in only 25% of cases.[34] Organisms derive from normal skin flora, soil contamination of the wound, or hospital pathogens acquired during medical interventions. The most commonly isolated pathogens include *S aureus*, coagulase-negative staphylococci, and aerobic gram-negative bacilli. A variety of other microbes including enterococci, anaerobes, fungi, and mycobacteria may be identified. In combat injuries, resistant strains of *Acinetobacter baumanii* and *P aeruginosa* have been implicated.[35] Flora are similar in adults and children.

Prevention of infection in traumatic fracture is comprehensively discussed in the article. Prompt debridement, surgical fixation, and local and systemic antimicrobial therapy are active considerations.

The clinical presentation of posttraumatic osteomyelitis is one of poor wound healing and fracture nonunion. Fever, wound drainage, warmth, pain, and erythema may occur. Diagnosis involves, as in other settings, a combination of clinical signs, laboratory markers, microbiology and histopathology from biopsy specimens, and imaging studies.[36] Microbiologic diagnosis does not occur the time of initial debridement, but rather at the time of debridement for possible subsequent infection.

Established osteomyelitis often warrants combined medical and surgical therapy. Fracture nonunion is managed by debridement and fixation as necessary. Bone and tissue cultures guide pathogen-directed antimicrobial therapy (see **Table 3**). Fixation hardware placed during active infection may need to be removed later after a course of antibiotics, with further debridement,[37] soft tissue coverage,[38] and antibiotics at that time as needed. When previously placed hardware cannot be removed, prolonged oral antibiotic suppression may be required after initial parenteral treatment for 4 to 6 weeks.

Osteomyelitis in Sickle Cell Disease

Bone and joint infections are recognized and common complications of sickle cell disease, occurring in more than 10% of patients.[17,39] Long bones are the most common sites of infection, occurring mostly in the pediatric and young adult age groups. Salmonella species and S aureus are the most commonly isolated pathogens.

Because bone pain owing to vasoocclusion, fever, and leukocytosis are common symptoms in sickle cell crisis, it can be difficult to confirm a diagnosis of infection. In 1 study in children, prolonged fever ($\geq$1 days) and pain (5 days) at presentation, as well as swelling of the affected limb, were signals of infection.[40] Plain radiographs are nonspecific for infection in sickle cell patients. Conversely, osteomyelitis was less common when more than 1 painful site was present. Nuclear radiology studies show normal uptake on bone marrow scan and abnormal uptake on bone scan at the painful site. CT-guided aspirate is used to obtain a microbiologic diagnosis, particularly when blood cultures are negative. Antibiotics should include coverage against S aureus and Salmonella in the empiric setting, with pathogen-directed therapy whenever possible (see **Table 3**).

Osteomyelitis and Injection Drug Use

In patients using injection drugs, organisms may seed the bones by 2 major routes, namely, hematogenous and inoculation.[41] The most common route is hematogenous, with a variety of joints and sometimes multiple joints potentially involved, including hips, knees, ankles, the sternoclavicular joints, and the spine. Endocarditis may be an intermediary in this process, with seeded heart valves secondarily infecting bone and joint sites. Because injection drug users access a number of different vascular sites, inoculation osteomyelitis may involve less common sites of infection. These include the clavicle and sternoclavicular joints, and the pubic symphysis. The most commonly isolated pathogens are also familiar as causes of endocarditis in this population: S aureus (especially methicillin-resistant strains), P aeruginosa, Eikenella corrodens, and Candida species. The treatment of osteomyelitis in this clinical setting is as described for other populations. Site of care and route of drug administration for outpatient care should be assessed carefully in these patients. Injection drug users have an increased risk of exposure to M tuberculosis, which can infect bone, especially in the thoracic spine.

Osteomyelitis and Hemodialysis

Patients undergoing hemodialysis require frequent access of the vascular tree. Although bloodstream infections are less common in patients using indwelling fistulas for access, they are relatively common in patients using vascular catheters for access. This places hemodialysis patients at risk for seeding of musculoskeletal sites, a risk that may be multiplied by diabetes mellitus, which is a common cause of end-stage renal disease.[42] S aureus, often methicillin-resistant, is the most common pathogen in multiple categories of infection of hemodialysis patients, including osteomyelitis. Coagulase-negative staphylococci, enterococci, aerobic gram-negative bacilli, and Candida species are also identified. Multiple sites may be seeded, including spine and large joints. Medical/surgical treatment of musculoskeletal infection in hemodialysis is as detailed for other patient populations.

Infections of the Bony Pelvis

Possible causes of pelvic osteomyelitis include hematogenous, pelvic trauma, or surgery. However, the most common source of infection of the bony pelvis is spread from a contiguous focus of infection in a chronic, stage IV decubitus ulcer to the sacral area.[43] In addition to ulceration, the clinical presentation may include erythema, induration, and fluctuance suggesting an underlying abscess. When there is an isolated, unstageable ulcer with eschar, the presence or absence of osteomyelitis is sometimes difficult to assess, given inability to view the bone. Leukocytosis and elevation of acute phase reactants such as erythrocyte sedimentation rate and C-reactive protein are helpful diagnostic adjuncts, but nonspecific. Plain radiographs are insensitive, and improved radiographic detail is obtained with cross-sectional imaging, with MRI studies preferred to CT scans. The microbiology of sacral osteomyelitis is often polymicrobial, given the proximity to the gastrointestinal flora. Swab cultures from the wound yield surface flora that are discordant with deep cultures. More accurate microbiologic data are obtained from deep bone and tissue cultures at the time of debridement. Adequate debridement to healthy bone with adjunct soft tissue coverage procedures is desirable and decreases the rate of readmission, but may be difficult with extensive disease. For this reason, chronic pelvic osteomyelitis, although frequently treatable with long courses (6–8 weeks intravenously) of broad-spectrum antibiotics, is often incurable. In such patients, the most common treatment algorithm involves partial debridement and treatment of flares with parenteral and oral antibiotics for defined courses.

Osteitis of the pubic symphysis arises most often as a complication of urologic[44] and gynecologic[45,46] surgery or hernia repairs, but has been identified in athletes with pelvic trauma[47,48] and in vaginal childbirth. It is not always an infectious disorder, but differentiating between the infectious and uninfected forms be challenging.[49,50] The pathophysiology of painful processes in this area seems to be heterogeneous, with some patients presenting with contiguous extension of abscess after surgery, and some with culture-negative osteitis without surgery. In the latter group, it has been postulated that injury to the blood supply or reflex sympathetic dystrophy may contribute to the disease. The presentation is subacute to chronic onset of pain in the pubic symphysis with a significant gait disorder. Because of the weight-bearing load on the pelvis, this entity may limit mobility severely. Fever is uncommon. Leukocytosis and acute phase reactant elevation may be absent or modest, and are nonspecific. Plain radiographs are often normal, and cross-sectional imaging such as CT scans or MRI studies offers more anatomic detail and helps to differentiate between osteitis and osteomyelitis. When these studies are unrevealing and the diagnosis is still suspected, white blood cell scanning may be helpful. Percutaneous or surgical biopsy offers the opportunity to confirm osteomyelitis at the site, but is reserved for patients where there is high clinical and radiographic suspicion. When present, microbiologic flora correspond with the underlying process, usually staphylococci, streptococci, enterococci, or aerobic gram-negative bacilli. Because surgical debridement carries significant morbidity, antibiotic therapy and conservative measures such as nonsteroidal antiinflammatory drugs are often a first line of treatment. Prolonged courses of intravenous antibiotics, usually in the range of 6 to 8 weeks, may be required for proven infection. Various durations of subsequent pathogen directed oral therapy have been used in clinical practice, although their role in this setting is not defined in the literature.

REFERENCES

1. Lew DP, Waldvogel FA. Osteomyelitis. Lancet 2004;364(9431):369–79.
2. Bryant T. A manual for the practice of surgery. 4th edition. Philadelphia: Henry C. Lea's Sons & Co; 1885. p. 917.
3. Lew DP, Waldvogel FA. Osteomyelitis. N Engl J Med 1997;336(14):999–1007.

4. Cierny G 3rd, Mader JT, Penninck JJ. A clinical staging system for adult osteomyelitis. Clin Orthop Relat Res 2003;(414):7–24.

5. Calhoun JH, Manring MM, Shirtliff M. Osteomyelitis of the long bones. Semin Plast Surg 2009;23(2):59–72.

6. Nathoo N, Caris EC, Wiener JA, et al. History of the vertebral venous plexus and the significant contributions of Breschet and Batson. Neurosurgery 2011;69(5): 1007–14 [discussion: 1014].

7. Patti JM, Allen BL, McGavin MJ, et al. MSCRAMM-mediated adherence of microorganisms to host tissues. Annu Rev Microbiol 1994;48:585–617.

8. Hudson MC, Ramp WK, Frankenburg KP. Staphylococcus aureus adhesion to bone matrix and bone-associated biomaterials. FEMS Microbiol Lett 1999; 173(2):279–84.

9. Mader JT, Ortiz M, Calhoun JH. Update on the diagnosis and management of osteomyelitis. Clin Podiatr Med Surg 1996;13(4):701–24.

10. Sarkissian EJ, Gans I, Gunderson MA, et al. Community-acquired methicillin-resistant staphylococcus aureus musculoskeletal infections: Emerging trends over the past decade. J Pediatr Orthop 2016;36(3):323–7.

11. Pigrau-Serrallach C, Rodriguez-Pardo D. Bone and joint tuberculosis. Eur Spine J 2013;22(Suppl 4):556–66.

12. Clavel G, Grados F, Lefauveau P, et al. Osteoarticular side effects of BCG therapy. Joint Bone Spine 2006;73(1):24–8.

13. Bariteau JT, Waryasz GR, McDonnell M, et al. Fungal osteomyelitis and septic arthritis. J Am Acad Orthop Surg 2014;22(6):390–401.

14. Medaris LA, Ponce B, Hyde Z, et al. Cryptococcal osteomyelitis: a report of 5 cases and a review of the recent literature. Mycoses 2016;59(6):334–42.

15. Blinkhorn RJ Jr, Strimbu V, Effron D, et al. 'Punch' actinomycosis causing osteomyelitis of the hand. Arch Intern Med 1988;148(12):2668–70.

16. Chelli Bouaziz M, Ladeb MF, Chakroun M, et al. Spinal brucellosis: a review. Skeletal Radiol 2008;37(9):785–90.

17. Aguilar C, Vichinsky E, Neumayr L. Bone and joint disease in sickle cell disease. Hematol Oncol Clin North Am 2005;19(5):929–41, viii.

18. McHenry MC, Easley KA, Locker GA. Vertebral osteomyelitis: long-term outcome for 253 patients from 7 Cleveland-area hospitals. Clin Infect Dis 2002;34(10): 1342–50.

19. Moenster RP, Linneman TW, Call WB, et al. The potential role of newer gram-positive antibiotics in the setting of osteomyelitis of adults. J Clin Pharm Ther 2013;38(2):89–96.

20. Selva Olid A, Sola I, Barajas-Nava LA, et al. Systemic antibiotics for treating diabetic foot infections. Cochrane Database Syst Rev 2015;(9):CD009061.

21. Peters EJ, Lipsky BA, Aragon-Sanchez J, et al. Interventions in the management of infection in the foot in diabetes: a systematic review. Diabetes Metab Res Rev 2016;32(Suppl 1):145–53.

22. Berendt AR, Peters EJ, Bakker K, et al. Diabetic foot osteomyelitis: a progress report on diagnosis and a systematic review of treatment. Diabetes Metab Res Rev 2008;24(Suppl 1):S145–61.

23. Gutierrez K. Bone and joint infections in children. Pediatr Clin North Am 2005; 52(3):779–94, vi.

24. Fernandez M, Carrol CL, Baker CJ. Discitis and vertebral osteomyelitis in children: an 18-year review. Pediatrics 2000;105(6):1299–304.

25. Wong M, Isaacs D, Howman-Giles R, et al. Clinical and diagnostic features of osteomyelitis occurring in the first three months of life. Pediatr Infect Dis J 1995;14(12):1047–53.

26. de Jesus LE, Fernandes A, Sias SM, et al. Neonatal osteomyelitis and complex nephro-ureteral duplication. Surg Infect (Larchmt) 2011;12(1):73–5.

27. Dartnell J, Ramachandran M, Katchburian M. Haematogenous acute and sub-acute paediatric osteomyelitis: a systematic review of the literature. J Bone Joint Surg Br 2012;94(5):584–95.

28. El Houmami N, Minodier P, Dubourg G, et al. Patterns of Kingella kingae disease outbreaks. Pediatr Infect Dis J 2016;35(3):340–6.

29. Ogden JA. Pediatric osteomyelitis and septic arthritis: the pathology of neonatal disease. Yale J Biol Med 1979;52(5):423–48.

30. Lam K, van Asten SA, Nguyen T, et al. Diagnostic accuracy of probe to bone to detect osteomyelitis in the diabetic foot: a systematic review. Clin Infect Dis 2016; 63(7):944–8.

31. Seabold JE, Flickinger FW, Kao SC, et al. Indium-111-leukocyte/technetium-99m-MDP bone and magnetic resonance imaging: difficulty of diagnosing osteomyelitis in patients with neuropathic osteoarthropathy. J Nucl Med 1990;31(5):549–56.

32. Lipsky BA, Berendt AR, Cornia PB, et al. 2012 Infectious Diseases Society of America clinical practice guideline for the diagnosis and treatment of diabetic foot infections. Clin Infect Dis 2012;54(12):e132–73.

33. Patzakis MJ, Wilkins J. Factors influencing infection rate in open fracture wounds. Clin Orthop Relat Res 1989;(243):36–40.

34. Merritt K. Factors increasing the risk of infection in patients with open fractures. J Trauma 1988;28(6):823–7.

35. Johnson EN, Burns TC, Hayda RA, et al. Infectious complications of open type III tibial fractures among combat casualties. Clin Infect Dis 2007;45(4):409–15.

36. Trampuz A, Zimmerli W. Diagnosis and treatment of infections associated with fracture-fixation devices. Injury 2006;37(Suppl 2):S59–66.

37. Meadows SE, Zuckerman JD, Koval KJ. Posttraumatic tibial osteomyelitis: diag-nosis, classification, and treatment. Bull Hosp Jt Dis 1993;52(2):11–6.

38. May JW Jr, Jupiter JB, Gallico GG 3rd, et al. Treatment of chronic traumatic bone wounds. microvascular free tissue transfer: a 13-year experience in 96 patients. Ann Surg 1991;214(3):241–50 [discussion: 250–2].

39. Vaishya R, Agarwal AK, Edomwonyi EO, et al. Musculoskeletal manifestations of sickle cell disease: a review. Cureus 2015;7(10):e358.

40. Berger E, Saunders N, Wang L, et al. Sickle cell disease in children: differenti-ating osteomyelitis from vaso-occlusive crisis. Arch Pediatr Adolesc Med 2009; 163(3):251–5.

41. Kak V, Chandrasekar PH. Bone and joint infections in injection drug users. Infect Dis Clin North Am 2002;16(3):681–95.

42. Lewis SS, Sexton DJ. Metastatic complications of bloodstream infections in he-modialysis patients. Semin Dial 2013;26(1):47–53.

43. Bodavula P, Liang SY, Wu J, et al. Pressure ulcer-related pelvic osteomyelitis: a neglected disease? Open Forum Infect Dis 2015;2(3):ofv112.

44. Kaplon DM, Iannotti H. Prostatic capsular perforation with extravasation resulting in pubic osteomyelitis: a rare complication of KTP laser prostatectomy. J Endourol 2008;22(12):2705–6.

45. Iavazzo C, Gkegkes ID. Osteomyelitis after robotically assisted laparoscopic sacral colpopexy. Acta Inform Med 2013;21(2):143.

46. Apostolis CA, Heiselman C. Sacral osteomyelitis after laparoscopic sacral colpopexy performed after a recent dental extraction: a case report. Female Pelvic Med Reconstr Surg 2014;20(6):e5–7.
47. Ukwu HN, Graham BS, Latham RH. Acute pubic osteomyelitis in athletes. Clin Infect Dis 1992;15(4):636–8.
48. Graham CW, Dmochowski RR, Faerber GJ, et al. Pubic osteomyelitis following bladder neck surgery using bone anchors: a report of 9 cases. J Urol 2002; 168(5):2055–7 [discussion: 2057–8].
49. Rosenthal RE, Spickard WA, Markham RD, et al. Osteomyelitis of the symphysis pubis: a separate disease from osteitis pubis. report of three cases and review of the literature. J Bone Joint Surg Am 1982;64(1):123–8.
50. Sexton DJ, Heskestad L, Lambeth WR, et al. Postoperative pubic osteomyelitis misdiagnosed as osteitis pubis: report of four cases and review. Clin Infect Dis 1993;17(4):695–700.

Prevention of Infection in Open Fractures

Charalampos G. Zalavras, MD, PhD, FACS

KEYWORDS

- Open fracture • Infection • Antibiotics • Debridement • Soft tissue coverage
- Fracture fixation

KEY POINTS

- Open fractures are challenging injuries and are associated with increased risk for complications, such as infection.
- The goals of open fracture management are prevention of infection, fracture union, and restoration of function.
- Management principles include careful patient and injury assessment, early administration of antibiotics, thorough surgical debridement, wound management with soft tissue coverage, and stable fracture fixation.

INTRODUCTION

Open fractures are often the result of high-energy trauma and may be associated with life-threatening injuries.[1] Open fractures are characterized by definition by soft tissue injury that results in communication of the fracture site with the outside environment and contamination of the fracture site with microorganisms or even introduction of foreign bodies into the wound.[2] Moreover, depending on the severity of injury, there is damage to the surrounding soft tissue envelope and to bone vascularity, which compromises the healing potential, as well as the response of the host defense mechanisms to contaminating microorganisms. As a result, open fractures are associated with increased risk for complications, such as infection and nonunion, and present a challenging problem to the treating physician.

The goals of open fracture management are prevention of infection, fracture union, and restoration of function. These goals are best achieved by careful patient and injury evaluation, early administration of systemic antibiotics supplemented by local delivery of antibiotics in severe injuries, thorough surgical debridement, wound management

Disclosure Statement: The author has nothing to disclose.
LAC+USC Medical Center, Keck School of Medicine, University of Southern California, 1200 North State Street, GNH 3900, Los Angeles, CA 90033, USA
E-mail address: zalavras@usc.edu

Infect Dis Clin N Am 31 (2017) 339–352
http://dx.doi.org/10.1016/j.idc.2017.01.005
0891-5520/17/© 2017 Elsevier Inc. All rights reserved.

with soft tissue coverage if needed, and stable fracture fixation. Key principles in prevention of infection following open fractures are summarized in **Box 1.**

EVALUATION AND CLASSIFICATION
Evaluation of Patient and Extremity

Open fractures are often caused by high-energy trauma, such as motor vehicle, motorcycle, and auto versus pedestrian injuries, and may be associated with potentially life-threatening injuries to the head, chest, and abdomen.[1,3] The injury severity score of patients with open diaphyseal fractures of the femur is 18.1 on average.[1] Thorough evaluation of every patient with an open fracture is necessary to diagnose and treat associated injuries, and appropriate resuscitation measures should be initiated on presentation of the patient.

The neurovascular status of the injured extremity should be carefully assessed and documented. The size, location, and degree of gross contamination of the open fracture wound should be evaluated. The wound should be irrigated, gross contamination should be removed, and a sterile dressing should be applied. The treating surgeon should not forget that the complication of compartment syndrome may still develop, despite the presence of the open fracture wound, especially in injuries with a severe crushing component.[4] The fractured extremity should be grossly realigned and immobilized with a splint. Intravenous antibiotic therapy should be started and tetanus prophylaxis should be given depending on the patient's immunization status. Fracture characteristics, such as location, articular involvement, and comminution, should be assessed by imaging studies to plan fixation of the fracture.

Classification of Open Fractures

Open fractures vary in severity depending on the mechanism and energy of injury. Therefore, classification systems of open fractures have been developed to describe the injury, guide treatment, determine prognosis, and compare various treatment methods for research purposes. The classification system of Gustilo and Anderson, subsequently modified by Gustilo, Mendoza, and Williams, has been extensively used (**Box 2**).[5,6] Newer classification systems have also been proposed.[7]

Box 1
Key principles in prevention of infection after open fractures

- Detailed evaluation of patient for associated and potentially life-threatening injuries.
- Systemic antibiotic therapy on patient presentation.
- Intraoperative assessment of severity of injury and classification of open fracture.
- Thorough surgical debridement with removal of all devitalized tissue and foreign bodies.
- Local antibiotic delivery with the bead-pouch technique in severe injuries.
- Primary wound closure is an option for less-severe injuries if only healthy, viable tissue is present in the wound after a meticulous debridement.
- Delayed closure with second-look debridement for more severe injuries.
- Local or free muscle flaps for extensive soft tissue damage.
- Fracture stabilization with appropriate technique based on fracture, soft tissue, and patient characteristics.

Box 2
Gustilo and Anderson classification of open fractures

- Type I: Wound of 1 cm or smaller, with minimal contamination or muscle crushing.

- Type II: Wound more than 1 cm long with moderate soft tissue damage and crushing. Bone coverage is adequate and comminution is minimal.

- Type IIIA: Extensive soft tissue damage, often due to a high-energy injury with a crushing component. Massively contaminated wounds and severely comminuted or segmental fractures are included in this subtype. Bone coverage is adequate.

- Type IIIB: Extensive soft tissue damage with periosteal stripping and bone exposure, usually with severe contamination and bone comminution. Flap coverage is required.

- Type IIIC: Arterial injury requiring repair.

The severity of the open fracture determines the risk of infection, which ranges from 0% to 2% for type I open fractures, 2% to 10% for Type II, and 10% to 50% for type III fractures.[6,8]

As with all classification systems, reliability of the classification and agreement among observers remains an issue. A study evaluating the responses of orthopedic surgeons who were asked to classify open fractures of the tibia on the basis of videotaped case presentations reported that the average agreement among observers was 60%.[9]

It is important to remember that the true extent and severity of the injury cannot be accurately assessed in the emergency department. The degree of contamination and soft tissue crushing are important factors for classifying an open fracture that may be mistakenly overlooked in a wound of small size. Therefore, classification of the fracture should be done in the operating room following wound exploration and debridement.

ANTIBIOTIC ADMINISTRATION

Early antibiotic administration is a key principle of open fracture management, because most patients with open fractures have wounds contaminated with microorganisms.[5,10] Systemic antibiotics should be administered in all patients with open fractures and local antibiotics in select cases.

Role of Antibiotics in Reducing Infection

The role of antibiotics in reducing the infection rate in patients with open fractures was demonstrated by Patzakis and colleagues[10] in a prospective randomized study. The infection rate when cephalothin was administered before debridement was 2.3% (2 of 84 fractures) compared with 13.9% (11 of 79 fractures) when no antibiotics were used.[10]

Timing of Antibiotics

Early antibiotic administration is very important. Patzakis and Wilkins[8] initially reported in 1989 that a delay longer than 3 hours from injury was associated with increased risk of infection. Subsequent animal and clinical studies have corroborated these findings. Penn-Barwell and colleagues[11] used a rat femur model with a defect contaminated with *Staphylococcus aureus* and found that delaying antibiotics to 6 or 24 hours had a detrimental effect on the infection rate regardless of the timing of surgery. Lack and colleagues[12] in a retrospective study of 137 type III open tibia factors demonstrated that administration of antibiotics beyond 66 minutes from injury was an independent risk factor for infection with an odds ratio of almost 4.

Choice of Antibiotics

Although the necessity of antibiotics has been definitively established, there is no consensus on the optimal choice of agents and specifically on the necessity of gram-negative coverage, especially for less-severe injuries.

In severe (type III) open fractures there is wide agreement that gram-positive and gram-negative coverage is needed and this is usually provided by a first-generation cephalosporin, such as cefazolin, and by an aminoglycoside, such as gentamicin.[8,13–16] However, others have advocated against aminoglycoside use and gram-negative coverage.[17]

In less-severe (type I and II) open fractures some investigators have recommended coverage only for gram-positive organisms with administration of a cephalosporin.[13–15] In contrast, combined gram-positive and gram-negative coverage for these less-severe open fractures has been proposed by other investigators to provide coverage against contaminating gram-negative organisms.[8,16]

Patzakis and Wilkins[8] reported that combination therapy in open tibia fractures reduced the infection rate (4.5%, 5 of 109) compared with cephalosporin only (13%, 25 of 192). This study did not analyze type I and II open fractures separately but the distribution of fracture types was comparable between the 2 groups that received combination therapy versus cephalosporin only.

It is important to remember that the severity of injury will be better appreciated in the operating room following wound exploration and debridement and an open fracture may be misclassified in the emergency department. As a result, a type IIIA open fracture with a wound of small size may be misclassified as type I or II open fracture and treated with cephalosporin only. Interestingly, a study of 189 patients with 202 open fractures, most of which were treated without gram-negative coverage, reported that gram-negative organisms were isolated in in 55% of the infections that developed during follow-up.[18]

The potential nephrotoxicity of aminoglycosides is a concern that may explain the reluctance to administer aminoglycosides in the setting of open fractures. A recent study evaluated patients with open fractures who were treated either with cefazolin (n = 41) or with cefazolin and gentamicin (n = 113).[19] Baseline characteristics and risk factors for renal dysfunction did not vary between groups. There was no difference in the development of acute kidney injury (4.8% in patients receiving cefazolin vs 4% patients receiving cefazolin and gentamicin).[19] This may be, in part, due to the short duration of aminoglycosides used.

Quinolones have been proposed as an oral alternative to intravenous antibiotics, based on their broad-spectrum antimicrobial coverage, bactericidal properties, oral administration, and good tolerance. A randomized prospective study showed that ciprofloxacin as a single agent in type I and II open fractures resulted in a similar infection rate (6%) compared with combination therapy with cefamandole and gentamicin.[20] However, in type III open fractures, ciprofloxacin was associated with a higher infection rate of 31% compared with 7.7% in the combination therapy group. Moreover, quinolones have been associated with inhibition of osteoblasts.[21] Quinolones are excellent agents against gram-negative pathogens and are considered an alternative when aminoglycosides cannot be used.

A recent study compared use of piperacillin/tazobactam versus cefazolin plus gentamicin for antibiotic prophylaxis in patients with type 3 open fractures and found similar rates of surgical site infections at 1 year (31.4% vs 32.4%, respectively).[22]

Piperacillin/tazobactam has a spectrum of activity similar to that of a cephalosporin plus an aminoglycoside, but its advantages include administration of a single agent and coverage against anaerobes in cases of fecal or clostridial contamination that may occur with farm-related injuries.

Anaerobic coverage (eg, penicillin, clindamycin, or metronidazole) should be added in injuries with potential contamination with clostridial organisms (eg, farm injuries) and in vascular injuries that can create conditions of ischemia and low oxygen tension. The goal is to prevent clostridial myonecrosis (gas gangrene). However, prevention of this catastrophic and life-threatening complication is primarily based on thorough surgical debridement. Antibiotic therapy is not a substitute for inadequate debridement.

Antimicrobial resistance in bacteria has been emerging and infections due to methicillin-resistant *S aureus* (MRSA), multidrug-resistant gram-negative bacilli, and vancomycin-resistant *Enterococci* are progressively increasing. This creates concerns about the adequacy of current antibiotic protocols, especially against MRSA. On the other hand, expanded prophylactic coverage with vancomycin may facilitate the emergence of glycopeptide-resistant organisms. A randomized controlled trial compared administration of a combination of vancomycin and cefazolin to administration of only cefazolin in 101 patients with open fractures and found no difference in the infection rates between the group receiving vancomycin and cefazolin (19%) versus the group receiving only cefazolin (15%).[23] As a result, the routine use of vancomycin in open fractures cannot be recommended based on available data. Antibiotic choices are summarized in **Table 1**.

The Role of Wound Cultures

Wound cultures obtained at patient presentation or intraoperatively do not help select the optimal antibiotic regimen, because they fail to identify the organism causing a subsequent infection in most cases.[24,25] Only 18% (3 of 17) of infections that developed in a series of 171 open fractures were caused by an organism identified by perioperative cultures.[20] Another study reported that predebridement cultures identified the infecting organism only 22% of the time and postdebridement cultures 42% of

Table 1 Choice of antibiotics in open fractures		
Severity of Open Fracture	**Proposed Coverage**	**Antibiotic Options**
Type I, II	• Gram-positive organisms (some investigators) OR • Gram-positive and gram-negative organisms (some investigators)	• Cephalosporin (1st generation) OR • Cephalosporin (1st generation) and aminoglycoside (quinolone as alternative for gram-negative coverage)
Type III	• Gram-positive and gram-negative organisms (some investigators)	• Cephalosporin (1st generation) and aminoglycoside (quinolone as alternative for gram-negative coverage) OR • Piperacillin/tazobactam
Potential contamination with clostridial organisms OR vascular injuries	• Additional coverage for anaerobic organisms	• Penicillin OR clindamycin OR metronidazole

the time.[25] Postdebridement cultures would be preferable to predebridement cultures to select the best agents in the case of an early infection, but their accuracy is still suboptimal. In most cases, infections are not caused by the organisms initially present in the wound but by nosocomial organisms that subsequently contaminate the wound.

Duration of Systemic Antibiotic Therapy

The optimal length of antibiotic therapy remains controversial. The recommended duration of antibiotic therapy is 3 days,[8,15] although a study comparing 1 day to 5 days of antibiotics reported similar infection rates and suggested that 1 day of antibiotics may be an option.[26] An additional 3-day administration of antibiotics is recommended for subsequent surgical procedures, such as repeat debridement and wound coverage.[8,15]

Local Antibiotic Therapy

Local delivery of antibiotic therapy used as an adjunct to systemic antibiotic therapy in the treatment of open fractures.[27] A commonly used delivery vehicle is polymethylmethacrylate (PMMA) cement, which can be manually molded by the surgeon to bead-resembling spheres with a diameter ranging from 5 to 10 mm or to spacer blocks of larger size. Bioabsorbable delivery vehicles, such as calcium sulfate, appear to be a promising alternative in clinical studies.[28] In a rat model of a contaminated bone defect, a bioabsorbable phospholipid gel resulted in lower infection rate compared with PMMA beads.[29]

An antibiotic appropriate for local delivery must be available in powder form because antibiotics in aqueous solution inhibit the polymerization process, must be heat stable to withstand the temperatures generated during the exothermic polymerization reaction, and should be active against the targeted microorganisms. Several antibiotics, including aminoglycosides, vancomycin, and cephalosporins, can be successfully incorporated into PMMA cement for local delivery. In open fractures, aminoglycosides are commonly used due to their broad spectrum of activity, heat stability, and low allergenicity.

The process of release of antibiotic from the delivery vehicle to the surrounding tissues is called elution. The difference in concentration of antibiotics between the delivery system and its environment is the key factor determining elution. Elution is facilitated by an increased surface-area–to-volume ratio of the delivery vehicle,[30] and by a high concentration of antibiotic in the beads or spacer.[31] The type of antibiotic plays a role and tobramycin has superior elution properties when compared with vancomycin.[32] A fluid medium is necessary for elution of antibiotics and the rate of fluid turnover influences the local antibiotic concentration. Elution of antibiotics from PMMA beads follows a biphasic pattern, with an initial rapid phase and a secondary slow phase.[33]

Antibiotic-impregnated PMMA beads are commercially available in Europe, but no similar product has been approved by the Food and Drug Administration for use in the United States. The delivery system has to be prepared in the operating room by the surgeon immediately before use. The PMMA powder is mixed with the antibiotic in powder form, is polymerized, and then formed into beads, which are incorporated on a 24-gauge wire. Usually 3.6 g of tobramycin are mixed with 40 g of PMMA cement. Antibiotic-impregnated PMMA beads are inserted in the open fracture wound, which is subsequently sealed by a semipermeable barrier so that the eluted antibiotic remains at the involved area to achieve a high local concentration.

The bead-pouch technique has unique advantages. First, it maintains antibiotics within the wound and achieves a high local concentration of antibiotics.[34] Second, the systemic concentration remains low, thus minimizing the adverse effects of aminoglycosides. The sealing of the wound from the external environment by the semipermeable barrier prevents secondary contamination by nosocomial pathogens and may safely extend the period for soft tissue transfers. At the same time, the semipermeable barrier establishes an aerobic wound environment, which is important for avoiding catastrophic anaerobic infections. Finally, it promotes patient comfort by avoiding painful dressing changes.

The antibiotic bead-pouch technique has been shown to reduce the infection rate when used in addition to systemic antibiotics for management of open fractures. Ostermann and colleagues[35] compared systemic antibiotics alone with combined treatment with both systemic antibiotics and the bead-pouch technique in a series of 1085 open fractures. The infection rate was considerably lower in the antibiotic bead-pouch group (3.7% [31 of 845 fractures] vs 12% [29 of 240 fractures]) but the reduction of infection was statistically significant in type III fractures only (6.5% for the antibiotic bead pouch vs 20.6% for systemic antibiotics alone).[35] A systematic review reported that the absolute rate of infection was lower for all types of open tibia fractures treated with intramedullary nailing when local antibiotics were administered in addition to systemic antibiotics.[36]

DEBRIDEMENT AND IRRIGATION
Debridement

Thorough surgical debridement plays a critical role in the management of open fractures.[37,38] Devitalized tissue and foreign material promote the growth of microorganisms, constitute a barrier for the host's defense mechanisms, and should be removed. Debridement should be performed in the operating room. Surgical extension of the wound allows assessment of the degree of soft tissue damage and contamination. Skin and subcutaneous tissue are sharply debrided back to bleeding edges. Muscle is debrided until bleeding is visualized. Viable muscle can be identified by its bleeding, color, and contractility. Bone fragments without soft tissue attachments are avascular and should be discarded. Articular fragments, however, should be preserved even if they have no attached blood supply, provided they are large enough and the surgeon believes reconstruction of the involved joint is possible. A repeat debridement can be performed after 24 to 48 hours based on the degree of contamination and soft tissue damage. The goal is a clean wound with viable tissues and no infection. In injuries requiring flap coverage, debridement should be also repeated at the time of the soft tissue procedure.

Timing of Debridement

Traditional concerns that delays in surgical management beyond 6 hours would lead to increased infection rates have not been substantiated in the literature.[8,39–43] Patzakis and Wilkins[8] reported in 1989 that the infection rate was similar in open fracture wounds debrided within 12 hours from injury (6.8%, 27 of 396) and in those debrided after 12 hours from injury (7.1%, 50 of 708) and concluded that elapsed time from injury to debridement is not a critical factor for development of infection in patients receiving antibiotic therapy.

Pollak and colleagues[40] and the LEAP study group found no relationship between time to surgical debridement and infection in 307 patients with severe open lower extremity fractures. The infection rate was 28%, 29%, and 26% in patients who underwent debridement earlier than 5 hours, 5 to 10 hours, and more than 10 hours from injury, respectively. Weber and colleagues,[43] in a prospective cohort study of 736 patients with open fractures, found no association between development of deep infection and time to debridement. In multivariate analysis, the only factors associated with infection were the severity (type III vs type I) and anatomic location (tibia vs upper extremity) of the fracture.

Although bacterial populations in an untreated contaminated wound increase over time, it appears that early antibiotic administration and thorough surgical debridement can effectively reduce the contamination present. As a result, small delays in surgical management do not appear to translate in increased infection rates and may allow for stabilization and resuscitation of the patient, as well as for treatment of the patient by experienced surgical teams with all necessary equipment available.

Irrigation

Irrigation mechanically removes foreign bodies and reduces the bacterial concentration.

Antiseptic solutions may be toxic to host cells and are better avoided.[44] A study comparing bacitracin solution to nonsterile castile soap solution for irrigation of open fractures found no difference in infection and nonunion rates, but an increased rate of wound-healing problems with bacitracin.[45] Irrigation with normal saline was not evaluated in this study.

High-pressure pulsatile lavage is more effective than low-pressure lavage in removing adherent bacteria if more than 6 hours have elapsed since the injury,[46] but it has been associated in experimental studies with bacterial seeding into the intramedullary canal,[46] with increased wound bacterial counts at 48 hours after irrigation,[47] and with adverse effects on early new bone formation.[48]

A recent randomized controlled trial of 2447 patients with open fractures compared the effects of different irrigation solutions (castile soap vs normal saline) and irrigation pressures (high pressure vs low pressure vs very low pressure) on the reoperation rate within 12 months from after the index surgery.[49] Irrigation with saline was associated with a significantly higher reoperation rate compared with castile soap (14.8% vs 11.6%). The reoperation rates were similar regardless of irrigation pressure, indicating that very low pressure (gravity) is an acceptable low-cost alternative method of irrigation.[49]

The author of the current article recommends irrigating the wound with 9 L of saline by gravity tubing.

WOUND MANAGEMENT
Wound Closure

The optimal time for wound closure remains controversial.[50] Primary wound closure generates concerns for potential development of the catastrophic complication of gas gangrene (clostridial myonecrosis) that may lead to loss of the limb or even death of the patient.[51] However, gas gangrene has mostly complicated military wounds with severe tissue injury, gross contamination, and inadequate antibiotic therapy or debridement.

Clinical studies of civilian injuries have not shown an increased infection rate following primary closure,[8,52–54] and suggested that primary closure may prevent secondary contamination and reduce surgical morbidity, hospital stay, and cost.[52,53] Patzakis and Wilkins[8] reported in 1989 that primary closure did not result in increased infection rate. Specifically, infection complicated 10.6% of wounds closed primarily compared with 13.4% of wounds closed with a delay.[8]

Primary closure of open fracture wounds is a viable option in carefully selected cases, provided there is no severe tissue damage and contamination, especially with soil or fecal matter, early administration of antibiotics has taken place, a meticulous debridement has been executed by an experienced surgeon, and the wound edges can be approximated without tension.

Partial wound closure is another option for less-severe injuries.[55] The surgical extension of the wound, created to assess the bone and soft tissues and facilitate debridement, can be closed primarily in type I and II open fractures, leaving only the injury wound open, to be closed in delayed fashion.

Delayed wound closure prevents anaerobic conditions in the wound, permits drainage, allows for repeat debridement at 24 to 48 hours, gives time to tissues of questionable viability to declare themselves, and facilitates use of the antibiotic bead-pouch technique. Delayed wound closure is recommended in injuries with extensive soft tissue damage and gross contamination, in patients presenting with a considerable delay, in wounds with tissues of questionable viability at the end of the debridement, and in wounds that cannot be approximated without tension.

If there is any doubt about the viability of the tissues and/or the adequacy of the debridement, the wound should not be closed primarily and a second-look debridement should be undertaken with the plan to perform delayed wound closure or a soft tissue coverage procedure, depending on the status of the soft tissue envelope.

In cases of delayed wound coverage, the wound should not be left exposed to the outside environment to prevent contamination with nosocomial pathogens. Instead, the antibiotic bead-pouch technique,[35] or negative-pressure wound therapy,[56] should be used.

Soft Tissue Reconstruction

When extensive damage to the soft tissues is present, as in type IIIB open fractures, adequate coverage may not be possible and soft tissue reconstruction is required. A well-vascularized soft tissue envelope promotes fracture healing, delivery of antibiotics, and action of the host defense mechanisms. It provides durable coverage, which prevents secondary contamination of the wound and desiccation of exposed anatomic structures, such as bone, cartilage, and tendons. The selection of coverage depends on the location and magnitude of the soft tissue defect.[57,58]

Soft tissue reconstruction is achieved with local or free tissue transfers. A microvascular surgeon should evaluate an open fracture with extensive soft tissue damage and participate in its management. Local pedicle muscle flaps include the gastrocnemius for proximal third tibia fractures and the soleus for middle third fractures. In distal third tibia fractures, free muscle flaps, such as the latissimus dorsi, the rectus abdominis, and the gracilis muscle, are necessary.[57,58] Free muscle flaps may be considered even in more proximally located fractures. Local muscles usually participate in the zone of injury; thus, their viability may be compromised. Pollak and colleagues[58] concluded that use of a free flap in limbs with a severe osseous injury was associated with fewer wound complications necessitating operative treatment compared with a rotational flap.

Soft tissue reconstruction should be performed early, within the first week from injury, because delays have been associated with increased flap and infectious complications.[12,24,59,60] Godina[60] advocated flap coverage within 72 hours. Gopal and colleagues[57] also used an early aggressive protocol in type IIIB and IIIC open fractures and observed deep infection in 6% (4/63) of fractures that were covered within 72 hours, compared with 29% (6/21) in fractures covered beyond 72 hours. It should be noted that in these studies the antibiotic bead pouch was not used, and therefore secondary contamination may have been an important confounding factor contributing to infectious complications.

FRACTURE FIXATION

Stabilization of the open fracture is an important part of management. Stability at the fracture site prevents further injury to the soft tissues, and enhances the host response to contaminating organisms.[61] In addition, fracture stability facilitates wound and patient care, and allows early motion and functional rehabilitation of the extremity. Fracture stabilization can be definitive or provisional and can be accomplished with intramedullary nailing, plate and screw fixation, or external fixation. Selection among these options depends on careful evaluation of fracture, soft tissue, and patient characteristics.[16] More than one method may be applicable to a specific injury and the surgeon's expertise and availability of implants should also be taken into account.

Intramedullary nailing is an effective method of stabilization of diaphyseal fractures of the lower extremity.[62,63] Statically interlocked intramedullary nailing maintains length and alignment of the fracture bone, is biomechanically superior to other methods, and does not interfere with soft tissue management. However, cortical circulation is disrupted to a variable degree, especially when reaming of the medullary canal takes place.[64] An animal study showed that, despite the adverse effect of reaming on endosteal perfusion, perfusion of callus and early strength of union were similar following intramedullary nailing with or without reaming.[65]

Plate and screw fixation is useful in intra-articular and metaphyseal fractures because it allows anatomic reduction and restoration of joint congruency.[66,67] Plate and screw fixation is recommended for open diaphyseal fractures of the forearm and humerus unless there is severe muscle damage and contamination.[68]

External fixation can be applied in a technically easy, safe, and expedient way, with minimal blood loss. For this reason, it can be beneficial in damage-control situations, such as type IIIC open fractures and unstable polytrauma patients.[69] External fixation preserves the vascularity of the fracture site and avoids implant insertion at the zone of injury. Therefore, it may be useful in wounds with severe soft tissue damage and gross contamination, as in type IIIB open fractures.[70,71] External fixation also can be useful as provisional joint-spanning fixation in open periarticular fractures followed by definitive fixation at a second stage.[72]

SUMMARY

Open fractures are challenging, often high-energy injuries that require a principle-based approach that starts with detailed evaluation of the patient for associated and potentially life-threatening injuries. The severity of the open fracture is best assessed intraoperatively and is an important factor in determining the rate of complications, such as infection and nonunion.

Systemic antibiotic therapy should be initiated on patient presentation. Local antibiotic delivery with the bead-pouch technique is beneficial in severe injuries.

Thorough surgical debridement with removal of all devitalized tissue and foreign bodies is critical for prevention of infection.

Primary wound closure is an option for less-severe injuries if only healthy, viable tissue is present in the wound after a meticulous debridement performed by an experienced surgeon. Delayed closure with a second-look debridement is recommended for more severe injuries. In the presence of extensive soft tissue damage, local or free muscle flaps should be transferred to achieve coverage. The open fracture should be stabilized using one of the available options based on fracture, soft tissue, and patient characteristics, and on surgeon's expertise. A management plan guided by the previously discussed principles will help prevent infection in these challenging injuries.

REFERENCES

1. Court-Brown CM, Bugler KE, Clement ND, et al. The epidemiology of open fractures in adults. A 15-year review. Injury 2012;43(6):891–7.
2. Zalavras CG, Patzakis MJ. Open fractures: evaluation and management. J Am Acad Orthop Surg 2003;11(3):212–9.
3. Gustilo RB. Management of open fractures. An analysis of 673 cases. Minn Med 1971;54(3):185–9.
4. Blick SS, Brumback RJ, Poka A, et al. Compartment syndrome in open tibial fractures. J Bone Joint Surg Am 1986;68(9):1348–53.
5. Gustilo RB, Anderson JT. Prevention of infection in the treatment of one thousand and twenty-five open fractures of long bones: retrospective and prospective analyses. J Bone Joint Surg Am 1976;58(4):453–8.
6. Gustilo RB, Mendoza RM, Williams DN. Problems in the management of type III (severe) open fractures: a new classification of type III open fractures. J Trauma 1984;24(8):742–6.
7. Evans AR, Agel J, Desilva GL. A new classification scheme for open fractures. J Orthop Trauma 2010;24(8):457–64.
8. Patzakis MJ, Wilkins J. Factors influencing infection rate in open fracture wounds. Clin Orthop Relat Res 1989;(243):36–40.
9. Brumback RJ, Jones AL. Interobserver agreement in the classification of open fractures of the tibia. The results of a survey of two hundred and forty-five orthopaedic surgeons. J Bone Joint Surg Am 1994;76(8):1162–6.
10. Patzakis MJ, Harvey JP Jr, Ivler D. The role of antibiotics in the management of open fractures. J Bone Joint Surg Am 1974;56(3):532–41.
11. Penn-Barwell JG, Murray CK, Wenke JC. Early antibiotics and debridement independently reduce infection in an open fracture model. J Bone Joint Surg Br 2012; 94(1):107–12.
12. Lack WD, Karunakar MA, Angerame MR, et al. Type III open tibia fractures: immediate antibiotic prophylaxis minimizes infection. J Orthop Trauma 2015; 29(1):1–6.
13. Hoff WS, Bonadies JA, Cachecho R, et al. East practice management guidelines work group: update to practice management guidelines for prophylactic antibiotic use in open fractures. J Trauma 2011;70(3):751–4.
14. Luchette FA, Bone LB, Born CT, et al. Practice management guidelines for prophylactic antibiotic use in open fractures. 2000. Available at. http://www.east. org/education/practice-management-guidelines/open-fractures-prophylactic-antibiotic-use-in-update.
15. Templeman DC, Gulli B, Tsukayama DT, et al. Update on the management of open fractures of the tibial shaft. Clin Orthop Relat Res 1998;(350):18–25.
16. Zalavras CG, Marcus RE, Levin LS, et al. Management of open fractures and subsequent complications. J Bone Joint Surg Am 2007;89(4):884–95.
17. Hauser CJ, Adams CA Jr, Eachempati SR, et al. Surgical Infection Society guideline: prophylactic antibiotic use in open fractures: an evidence-based guideline. Surg Infect (Larchmt) 2006;7(4):379–405.
18. Chen AF, Schreiber VM, Washington W, et al. What is the rate of methicillin-resistant *Staphylococcus aureus* and Gram-negative infections in open fractures? Clin Orthop Relat Res 2013;471(10):3135–40.
19. Pannell WC, Banks K, Hahn J, et al. Antibiotic related acute kidney injury in patients treated for open fractures. Injury 2016;47(3):653–7.

20. Patzakis MJ, Bains RS, Lee J, et al. Prospective, randomized, double-blind study comparing single-agent antibiotic therapy, ciprofloxacin, to combination antibiotic therapy in open fracture wounds. J Orthop Trauma 2000;14(8):529–33.

21. Holtom PD, Pavkovic SA, Bravos PD, et al. Inhibitory effects of the quinolone antibiotics trovafloxacin, ciprofloxacin, and levofloxacin on osteoblastic cells in vitro. J Orthop Res 2000;18:721–7.

22. Redfern J, Wasilko SM, Groth ME, et al. Surgical site infections in patients with type 3 open fractures: comparing antibiotic prophylaxis with cefazolin plus gentamicin versus piperacillin/tazobactam. J Orthop Trauma 2016;30(8):415–9.

23. Saveli CC, Morgan SJ, Belknap RW, et al. Prophylactic antibiotics in open fractures: a pilot randomized clinical safety study. J Orthop Trauma 2013;27(10): 552–7.

24. Fischer MD, Gustilo RB, Varecka TF. The timing of flap coverage, bone-grafting, and intramedullary nailing in patients who have a fracture of the tibial shaft with extensive soft-tissue injury. J Bone Joint Surg Am 1991;73(9):1316–22.

25. Lee J. Efficacy of cultures in the management of open fractures. Clin Orthop Relat Res 1997;(339):71–5.

26. Dellinger EP, Caplan ES, Weaver LD, et al. Duration of preventive antibiotic administration for open extremity fractures. Arch Surg 1988;123(3):333–9.

27. Zalavras CG, Patzakis MJ, Holtom P. Local antibiotic therapy in the treatment of open fractures and osteomyelitis. Clin Orthop Relat Res 2004;(427):86–93.

28. McKee MD, Wild LM, Schemitsch EH, et al. The use of an antibiotic-impregnated, osteoconductive, bioabsorbable bone substitute in the treatment of infected long bone defects: early results of a prospective trial. J Orthop Trauma 2002;16(9): 622–7.

29. Penn-Barwell JG, Murray CK, Wenke JC. Local antibiotic delivery by a bioabsorbable gel is superior to PMMA bead depot in reducing infection in an open fracture model. J Orthop Trauma 2014;28(6):370–5.

30. Holtom PD, Warren CA, Greene NW, et al. Relation of surface area to in vitro elution characteristics of vancomycin-impregnated polymethylmethacrylate spacers. Am J Orthop 1998;27:207–10.

31. Baker AS, Greenham LW. Release of gentamicin from acrylic bone cement. Elution and diffusion studies. J Bone Joint Surg Am 1988;70(10):1551–7.

32. Greene N, Holtom PD, Warren CA, et al. In vitro elution of tobramycin and vancomycin polymethylmethacrylate beads and spacers from simplex and palacos. Am J Orthop 1998;27(3):201–5.

33. Torholm C, Lidgren L, Lindberg L, et al. Total hip joint arthroplasty with gentamicin-impregnated cement. A clinical study of gentamicin excretion kinetics. Clin Orthop Relat Res 1983;(181):99–106.

34. Adams K, Couch L, Cierny G, et al. In vitro and in vivo evaluation of antibiotic diffusion from antibiotic-impregnated polymethylmethacrylate beads. Clin Orthop Relat Res 1992;(278):244–52.

35. Ostermann PA, Seligson D, Henry SL. Local antibiotic therapy for severe open fractures. A review of 1085 consecutive cases. J Bone Joint Surg Br 1995; 77(1):93–7.

36. Craig J, Fuchs T, Jenks M, et al. Systematic review and meta-analysis of the additional benefit of local prophylactic antibiotic therapy for infection rates in open tibia fractures treated with intramedullary nailing. Int Orthop 2014;38(5):1025–30.

37. Tetsworth K, Cierny G 3rd. Osteomyelitis debridement techniques. Clin Orthop Relat Res 1999;(360):87–96.

38. Swiontkowski MF. Criteria for bone debridement in massive lower limb trauma. Clin Orthop Relat Res 1989;(243):41–7.
39. Harley BJ, Beaupre LA, Jones CA, et al. The effect of time to definitive treatment on the rate of nonunion and infection in open fractures. J Orthop Trauma 2002; 16(7):484–90.
40. Pollak AN, Jones AL, Castillo RC, et al. The relationship between time to surgical debridement and incidence of infection after open high-energy lower extremity trauma. J Bone Joint Surg Am 2010;92(1):7–15.
41. Schenker ML, Yannascoli S, Baldwin KD, et al. Does timing to operative debridement affect infectious complications in open long-bone fractures? A systematic review. J Bone Joint Surg Am 2012;94(12):1057–64.
42. Skaggs DL, Friend L, Alman B, et al. The effect of surgical delay on acute infection following 554 open fractures in children. J Bone Joint Surg Am 2005;87(1): 8–12.
43. Weber D, Dulai SK, Bergman J, et al. Time to initial operative treatment following open fracture does not impact development of deep infection: a prospective cohort study of 736 subjects. J Orthop Trauma 2014;28(11):613–9.
44. Bhandari M, Adili A, Schemitsch EH. The efficacy of low-pressure lavage with different irrigating solutions to remove adherent bacteria from bone. J Bone Joint Surg Am 2001;83(3):412–9.
45. Anglen JO. Comparison of soap and antibiotic solutions for irrigation of lower-limb open fracture wounds. A prospective, randomized study. J Bone Joint Surg Am 2005;87(7):1415–22.
46. Bhandari M, Adili A, Lachowski RJ. High pressure pulsatile lavage of contaminated human tibiae: an in vitro study. J Orthop Trauma 1998;12(7):479–84.
47. Owens BD, White DW, Wenke JC. Comparison of irrigation solutions and devices in a contaminated musculoskeletal wound survival model. J Bone Joint Surg Am 2009;91(1):92–8.
48. Dirschl DR, Duff GP, Dahners LE, et al. High pressure pulsatile lavage irrigation of intraarticular fractures: effects on fracture healing. J Orthop Trauma 1998;12(7): 460–3.
49. FLOW Investigators, Bhandari M, Jeray KJ, et al. A trial of wound irrigation in the initial management of open fracture wounds. N Engl J Med 2015;373(27): 2629–41.
50. Weitz-Marshall AD, Bosse MJ. Timing of closure of open fractures. J Am Acad Orthop Surg 2002;10(6):379–84.
51. Patzakis MJ. Clostridial myonecrosis. Instr Course Lect 1990;39:491–3.
52. DeLong WG Jr, Born CT, Wei SY, et al. Aggressive treatment of 119 open fracture wounds. J Trauma 1999;46(6):1049–54.
53. Jenkinson RJ, Kiss A, Johnson S, et al. Delayed wound closure increases deep-infection rate associated with lower-grade open fractures: a propensity-matched cohort study. J Bone Joint Surg Am 2014;96(5):380–6.
54. Hohmann E, Tetsworth K, Radziejowski MJ, et al. Comparison of delayed and primary wound closure in the treatment of open tibial fractures. Arch Orthop Trauma Surg 2007;127(2):131–6.
55. Patzakis MJ, Wilkins J, Moore TM. Considerations in reducing the infection rate in open tibial fractures. Clin Orthop Relat Res 1983;(178):36–41.
56. Stannard JP, Volgas DA, Stewart R, et al. Negative pressure wound therapy after severe open fractures: a prospective randomized study. J Orthop Trauma 2009; 23(8):552–7.

57. Gopal S, Majumder S, Batchelor AG, et al. Fix and flap: the radical orthopaedic and plastic treatment of severe open fractures of the tibia. J Bone Joint Surg Br 2000;82(7):959–66.
58. Pollak AN, McCarthy ML, Burgess AR. Short-term wound complications after application of flaps for coverage of traumatic soft-tissue defects about the tibia. The Lower Extremity Assessment Project (LEAP) Study Group. J Bone Joint Surg Am 2000;82-A(12):1681–91.
59. Cierny G 3rd, Byrd HS, Jones RE. Primary versus delayed soft tissue coverage for severe open tibial fractures. A comparison of results. Clin Orthop Relat Res 1983;(178):54–63.
60. Godina M. Early microsurgical reconstruction of complex trauma of the extremities. Plast Reconstr Surg 1986;78(3):285–92.
61. Worlock P, Slack R, Harvey L, et al. The prevention of infection in open fractures: an experimental study of the effect of fracture stability. Injury 1994;25(1):31–8.
62. Brumback RJ, Ellison PS Jr, Poka A, et al. Intramedullary nailing of open fractures of the femoral shaft. J Bone Joint Surg Am 1989;71(9):1324–31.
63. Bhandari M, Guyatt G, Tornetta P 3rd, et al. Randomized trial of reamed and unreamed intramedullary nailing of tibial shaft fractures. J Bone Joint Surg Am 2008; 90(12):2567–78.
64. Schemitsch EH, Kowalski MJ, Swiontkowski MF, et al. Cortical bone blood flow in reamed and unreamed locked intramedullary nailing: a fractured tibia model in sheep. J Orthop Trauma 1994;8(5):373–82.
65. Schemitsch EH, Kowalski MJ, Swiontkowski MF, et al. Comparison of the effect of reamed and unreamed locked intramedullary nailing on blood flow in the callus and strength of union following fracture of the sheep tibia. J Orthop Res 1995; 13(3):382–9.
66. Benirschke SK, Agnew SG, Mayo KA, et al. Immediate internal fixation of open, complex tibial plateau fractures: treatment by a standard protocol. J Orthop Trauma 1992;6(1):78–86.
67. Kregor PJ, Stannard JA, Zlowodzki M, et al. Treatment of distal femur fractures using the less invasive stabilization system: surgical experience and early clinical results in 103 fractures. J Orthop Trauma 2004;18(8):509–20.
68. Moed BR, Kellam JF, Foster RJ, et al. Immediate internal fixation of open fractures of the diaphysis of the forearm. J Bone Joint Surg Am 1986;68(7):1008–17.
69. Pape HC, Tornetta P 3rd, Tarkin I, et al. Timing of fracture fixation in multitrauma patients: the role of early total care and damage control surgery. J Am Acad Orthop Surg 2009;17(9):541–9.
70. Edwards CC, Simmons SC, Browner BD, et al. Severe open tibial fractures. Results treating 202 injuries with external fixation. Clin Orthop Relat Res 1988;(230):98–115.
71. Marsh JL, Nepola JV, Wuest TK, et al. Unilateral external fixation until healing with the dynamic axial fixator for severe open tibial fractures. J Orthop Trauma 1991; 5(3):341–8.
72. Sirkin M, Sanders R, DiPasquale T, et al. A staged protocol for soft tissue management in the treatment of complex pilon fractures. J Orthop Trauma 1999; 13(2):78–84.

Fungal Musculoskeletal Infections

Michael W. Henry, MD[a], Andy O. Miller, MD[a], Thomas J. Walsh, MD[a,b,c],
Barry D. Brause, MD[a],*

KEYWORDS

- Fungi • Osteomyelitis • Septic arthritis • Prosthetic joint infection • Candida
- Aspergillus

KEY POINTS

- Fungal osteoarticular infections are complex infections that are seldom encountered in routine clinical practice.
- The clinical presentation is often subacute and diagnosis requires a high index of suspicion.
- Delayed diagnosis can lead to considerable morbidity.
- The treatment approach depends on the type of fungus present, the immune status of the host, the presence of foreign bodies, and the site of the infection.

INTRODUCTION

Fungal osteoarticular infections (OAI) are unusual but often destructive infections requiring surgery and prolonged antifungal therapy. These infections involve bone, joints, muscle, and connective tissue, such as ligaments and tendons, and can involve contiguous structures. The severity of these infections is related to the immune function of the host, the presence of foreign bodies, and the inherent pathogenicity of the organism. Over the past decade, there have been increasing reports of fungal musculoskeletal infections in both immunocompromised and immunocompetent hosts.[1]

PATHOGENESIS AND PRESENTATION

Fungal OAIs are caused by a wide variety of commensal, zoonotic, and environmental yeasts and molds. Although most of these infections occur in immunocompromised

Disclosure: Dr T.J. Walsh has received research grants in mycological research from Astellas, Pfizer, Merck, and Novartis. He has served as consultant to Astellas, Pfizer, Novartis, and Methylgene. The other authors have nothing to disclose.
[a] Division of Infectious Diseases, Department of Medicine, Hospital for Special Surgery, Weill Cornell Medicine, 535 East 70th Street, New York, NY 10021, USA; [b] Department of Pediatrics, Weill Cornell Medicine, 1300 York Avenue, New York, NY 10065, USA; [c] Department of Microbiology & Immunology, Weill Cornell Medicine, 1300 York Avenue, New York, NY 10065, USA
* Corresponding author.
E-mail address: brauseb@hss.edu

Infect Dis Clin N Am 31 (2017) 353–368
http://dx.doi.org/10.1016/j.idc.2017.01.006
0891-5520/17/© 2017 Elsevier Inc. All rights reserved.

hosts, healthy hosts can also develop these infections as well. *De novo* infections in immunocompetent hosts with environmental dimorphic fungi, such as *Coccidioides immitis* and *Blastomyces dermatitidis*, arise following hematogenous spread from their site of entry or via direct inoculation.[2] Healthy hosts can also develop fungal musculoskeletal infections from nosocomial exposures, such as prior surgery or placement of indwelling foreign bodies. Fungal infections can be introduced via direct implantation, as seen in the intravenous drug use community, in trauma victims, and as a complication of parenteral treatment, such as was seen with the recent *Exserohilum rostratum* outbreak in the United States, which stemmed from the contamination of preservative-free steroids used for local spinal or paraspinal injections.[3] Immunocompromised patients are susceptible to a wide range of yeast and mold musculoskeletal infections, both endogenous and from the environment. The mostly commonly reported genera are *Candida* and *Aspergillus*, but a wide array of other opportunistic fungi, including *Fusarium* spp, *Scedosporium* spp, Mucorales, and dematiaceous molds, have been reported.[4]

The basic underlying pathophysiology of fungal musculoskeletal infections mirrors that of more common bacterial infections. These infections can occur in isolation or as part of a systemic infection with multiple organ involvement. The site of infection can be reached hematogenously, by contiguous spread or by direct inoculation.[5,6] In the setting of hematogenous spread, involvement of more than 1 noncontiguous bone or joint is common. Any bone or joint can be a site of infection, although the large, weight-bearing joints and bones, vertebrae, and ribs are most commonly involved.[2,5,6] Contiguous spread can occur from adjacent bone or joints, as well as from infected soft tissue in close proximity, as is seen in skull-base osteomyelitis in the setting of untreated otogenic infections[7] or in the setting of eumycetoma.[8] Infection can also be introduced at the time of surgery. Given the delayed onset of infection in many cases, taking a careful history of prior procedures, including intra-articular injections, and of penetrating trauma to the site of infection, can help establish a route of direct inoculation. Increasingly, invasive fungal infections related to trauma sustained in combat or in natural disasters have been reported.[9,10] Many medically important fungi, including *Candida*, *Aspergillus*, *Cryptococcus*, *Coccidioides*, and *Trichosporon*, have been shown to form biofilm, which decreases the efficacy of antifungal treatment and may lead to intractable infections.[11,12]

Owing to their rarity and generally subacute presentation, the most important aspect of the diagnosis of these infections is their inclusion in the differential diagnosis, particularly in immunocompetent patients. Microbiologic and histologic detection of fungal infections can require specialized culture media and stains, which may not be used routinely during evaluation for an osteoarticular infection. Diagnoses can be delayed when positive cultures are assumed to be contaminants. Fungal OAI can present in a broad array symptoms and time of onset, depending on the pathogenicity of the underlying organism, the site of infection, and the underlying health of the patient. Local pain, swelling, and other typical signs of inflammation are the most common presenting symptoms and signs; with chronicity, sinus drainage and extension into soft tissue may develop.[6,13] These infections can mimic other processes, including malignancy, tuberculosis, and more routine bacterial infections.[14]

TREATMENT

The overall approach to treatment involves surgical debridement of necrotic and nonviable tissues, in combination with prolonged courses of antifungal therapy. In addition to debridement, surgical management also involves irrigation, removal of infected hardware when possible, fixation and/or grafting of bone, and use of antifungal-impregnated local depot materials, such as polymethyl methacrylate (PMMA) or calcium sulfate, to deliver high concentrations of antifungal agents into the immediate vicinity of the infection.[15] When possible, the immune status of the patient should be assessed and optimized. Although some infections can be cured with antifungal treatment alone,[2] a successful outcome can be difficult to achieve in the absence of surgical debridement, especially when infected orthopedic hardware or necrotic tissue is present. Antifungal treatment is guided by the identification and antifungal susceptibilities of the pathogen. There are several treatment guidelines addressing various fungal infections that include guidance for bone and joint infections[16–22] (**Table 1**). When an immunosuppressed state persists after initial treatment of the infection or when an infected foreign body cannot be removed, chronic prophylaxis or suppression may be used to prevent relapse or recrudescence.[16,21]

CANDIDA

The most common fungal group causing OAI, the ubiquitous saprophytic genus *Candida*, comprises at least 15 distinct species, of which *Candida albicans* is by far the most common. As immunosuppression and antifungal exposure increase, the incidence of infections caused by non-*albicans Candida* spp increases. Although some manifestations of candidiasis, such as mucosal infections, are ubiquitous in clinical practice, *Candida* OAIs are rare. Nevertheless, they comprise most fungal OAIs.

Although less frequent than *C albicans*, *Candida parapsilosis* may be overrepresented in OAI, perhaps because of its propensity for biofilm formation.[23–25] Optimal therapy for *C parapsilosis* remains an unsettled question in the absence of controlled clinical efficacy data. In vitro models suggest that echinocandins may offer enhanced activity (relative to azoles), despite increased minimum inhibitory concentrations of planktonic forms of *C parapsilosis* (relative to *C albicans*).[23,26–28] *Candida auris*, an emerging multidrug-resistant fungal pathogen initially described in Asia, causes invasive health care–associated infections. Isolates with increased minimum inhibitory concentrations against azoles, echinocandins, and polyenes have been described; this organism may pose a particular public health threat.[29,30] Although *C auris* has been described as a cause of diabetic foot infection,[31] other OAIs caused by this organism have not yet been described.

Choice of an empirical antifungal agent early in the diagnosis of candida OAI depends on the likelihood of antifungal drug resistance. There are growing data supporting the use of echinocandins in the treatment of candida OAI, although fluconazole remains the most commonly used agent for susceptible isolates.[32] Echinocandins, as well as liposomal amphotericin B, may hold particular promise against biofilms formed by multiple *Candida* species.[23,33]

Candida Osteomyelitis

Adult infections tend to involve the axial skeleton, whereas children have more long bone involvement.[6] Most cases occur in non-neutropenic hosts, and typically present with 2 or more sites of infection. Candidemia frequently precedes OAI, with a wide range in time to presentation and diagnosis.[34] Prior abdominal surgery, recent receipt of antibiotics, and intravenous access via central line or illicit drug use are important comorbidities of both candidemia and OAI.[34] Most patients are treated with surgery and antifungal therapy, and relapse is common, occurring in 32% of cases in the recent analysis of published literature.[6] The most common cause for relapse seems to be an initially inadequate length of therapy. Infectious Diseases Society of America (IDSA) guidelines recommend 6 to 12 months of fluconazole, with or without an initial echinocandin use, as initial therapy for candida osteomyelitis.[19]

Table 1
Summary of Infectious Diseases Society of America guidelines for the treatment of fungal osteoarticular infections

	Treatment	Comments
Candida sp	Fluconazole, or Echinocandin (caspofungin, micafungin, or anidulafungin) for at least 2 wk followed by fluconazole, or Liposomal AmB for at least 2 wk followed by fluconazole	Choice of antifungal agent should be guided by susceptibility testing Duration of treatment: Septic arthritis: 6 wk Osteomyelitis: 6–12 mo for osteomyelitis
Aspergillus sp	Primary: voriconazole Alternative: liposomal AmB Salvage: ABLC Caspofungin Micafungin Posaconazole Itraconazole	Duration: minimum of 8 wk, to >6 mo Guidelines recommend following same treatment protocols described for invasive pulmonary aspergillosis, but note that there is little experience with echinocandins in the treatment of aspergillus OAI
Cryptococcus neoformans	Osteoarticular infections are not specifically addressed in current IDSA guidelines Recommendations for extrapulmonary non-CNS cryptococcosis in immunocompetent patients: follow treatment protocol for CNS disease (see guidelines for separate recommendations for HIV-positive patients and for transplant recipients) Induction therapy: 1. AmB plus flucytosine for 4 wk 2. AmB for 6 wk 3. Liposomal AmB or ABLC combined with flucytosine, if possible, for 4 wk; or 4. AmB plus flucytosine for 2 wk (for patients at low risk for therapeutic failure; see guidelines) Consolidation therapy: fluconazole (400–800 mg/d) for 8 wk Maintenance therapy: fluconazole (200 mg/d) for 6–12 mo Patients without cryptococcemia and with a single site of infection and no immunosuppressive risk factors: Fluconazole for 6–12 mo Depending on immune status, patients may require long-term secondary prophylaxis with fluconazole	
C immitis	Mild-moderate disease: fluconazole or itraconazole Severe disease: liposomal AmB for 3 mo followed by fluconazole or itraconazole	Duration of therapy: 3 y to lifelong
Histoplasma capsulatum	Mild-moderate disease: itraconazole Severe disease: liposomal AmB for 2–6 wk, followed by itraconazole	Histoplasma osteoarticular infections usually occur in the setting of disseminated disease. Duration of therapy for disseminated disease: at least 12 mo
B dermatitidis	Mild-moderate disease: itraconazole Severe disease: liposomal AmB for 2 wk followed by itraconazole	Recommended duration of therapy for osteoarticular disease: at least 12 mo

(continued on next page)

Table 1 (continued)		
	Treatment	**Comments**
Sporothrix schenckii	Preferred: itraconazole Alternative: liposomal AmB with change to itraconazole after a favorable response is achieved	Recommended duration of therapy for osteoarticular disease: at least 12 mo

Please refer to Infectious Diseases Society of America guidelines for specific dosing recommendations.

Abbreviations: ABLC, amphotericin B lipid complex; AmB, amphotericin B; CNS, central nervous system; HIV, human immunodeficiency virus; IDSA, Infectious Diseases Society of America.

Data from Refs.[16–22]

Candida Septic Arthritis

Most patients with candida arthritis are not immunosuppressed, and knees represent 75% of cases. Adjacent osteomyelitis is frequent, and surgical approaches to treatment accompany antifungal use in most cases.[25] The duration of therapy for candida arthritis is not well defined. IDSA guidelines recommend surgical drainage and 6 weeks of fluconazole, with or without an initial echinocandin use, as initial therapy for candida septic arthritis.[19] However, a recent systematic review of candida arthritis found that the median duration of therapy was 64 days (range, 14–436 days).[24] There is substantial risk of relapse despite optimal surgical and medical therapy.[25]

ASPERGILLUS

Invasive aspergillosis, a major cause of fungal illness among immunocompromised patients, preferentially affects the respiratory and central nervous systems, and *Aspergillus* OAI often arises in local contiguity. *Aspergillus fumigatus*, *Aspergillus flavus*, and *Aspergillus nidulans* are the most commonly identified species that cause osteomyelitis.[35] Although immune impairment is a major risk factor, a substantial proportion of infected patients are immunocompetent.[5,36] Children with chronic granulomatous disease represent a high proportion of pediatric patients with aspergillus OAI.[5] Most cases present with multiple lesions, predominantly of the axial skeleton. Routes of infection may be hematogenous or contiguous; the predominant axial location of these infections may reflect their preference for vascular host tissues, or their contiguity with infected pulmonary parenchyma. Direct inoculation is unusual, especially among children,[5] but such infections are described following trauma and surgery.

Aspergillus Osteomyelitis

Aspergillus osteomyelitis predominantly affects the vertebrae, usually with associated spondylodiscitis and neurologic deficit; rib infection is significantly more likely in pediatric populations.[5] Cranial osteomyelitis can be a sequela of contiguous malignant otitis externa, and can arise in patients with diabetes, neutropenia, and other immune deficits. IDSA guidelines recommend surgical debridement and from 8 weeks to more than 6 months of voriconazole as initial therapy for aspergillus osteomyelitis.[20] Relapse rates are substantially higher in patients who are treated without surgery (30% vs 8%). Combination antifungal therapy does not seem to be of benefit in patients undergoing surgical debridement.[5]

Aspergillus Septic Arthritis

Aspergillus arthritis often arises in the setting of disseminated infection and in contiguity with osteomyelitis, but hematogenous, surgical, injection, and traumatic sources have been reported. Among adults, septic arthritis of the extremities is rare. IDSA guidelines recommend drainage, surgical debridement, and voriconazole, with or without an initial echinocandin use, as initial therapy for aspergillus septic arthritis.[20] Postoperative septic arthritis is an uncommon but potentially serious complication of elective orthopedic surgery.[37]

NON-*ASPERGILLUS* FILAMENTOUS FUNGI

OAI caused by the diverse non-*Aspergillus* molds, including *Fusarium* spp, *Scedosporium* spp, and *Rhizopus* spp, are uncommon but often severe, resulting either from direct inoculation from trauma or puncture (in approximately 50%) or from surgery, and are associated with severe underlying immunosuppression in approximately 62% of cases. Reports of such infections have increased over time.[4] Anatomic distribution is diverse; septic arthritis caused by these organisms is usually accompanied by osteomyelitis. Fever, increased levels of inflammatory markers, lower-limb involvement, and trauma are more common among children. Combination antifungal chemotherapy and surgical management remain the general mode of treatment, with a priority placed on the identification of the species (by culture) because susceptibility to antifungal agents varies considerably.[4,38,39]

A 2012 multistate outbreak of *E rostratum* central nervous system (CNS) infections and OAI in patients receiving epidural and intra-articular injections with contaminated methylprednisolone from a single source led to increased regulation and oversight of compounding pharmacies, and to a better understanding of the natural history, morbidity, diagnosis, and treatment of these rare infections.[3] Six months of voriconazole, with serum monitoring for adequate antifungal drug levels, emerged as a preferred chemotherapeutic regimen in patients with osteoarticular manifestations of disease, which included vertebral osteomyelitis and spondylodiscitis.[40]

Mycetoma may be caused by bacteria or fungi. The fungal-related (eumycotic) mycetoma or eumycetoma is a neglected major fungal infection in many tropical and subtropical regions that presents as an insidiously progressive disease involving skin, muscle, tendon, and bone.[41] Most frequently presenting as a chronic infection of the lower extremities (Madura foot) of young adult men, the disease is probably established by repeated traumatic inoculation. The most common cause of eumycotic mycetoma in temperate climates is *Scedosporium apiospermum*, whereas *Madurella mycetomatis*, *Streptomyces somaliensis*, and other species occur in subtropical and tropical regions. *S apiospermum*, which may be resistant to 1 or more antifungal agents, may be recognized in culture by characteristic conidia (annelloconidia) and by the sexual stage characterized as cleistothecia.[38]

As the mycetoma progresses, bony changes consistent with osteomyelitis and osteoporosis develop. Diagnostic imaging and pathology may show periosteal reaction, bony destruction, and other changes consistent with osteomyelitis. A large study suggested that the rate of cure among patients with eumycetoma was 25% among patients who remain in care, with more than 50% of patients lost to follow-up.[42] A combination of surgical and medical therapy is usually necessary; itraconazole and voriconazole are commonly used when available.[41]

CRYPTOCOCCUS

Cryptococcal OAI is rare, and is generally likely to be a manifestation of disseminated disease, even if no other signs and symptoms exist. Single circumscribed vertebral lesions are the most common; septic arthritis most commonly involves the knee.[43,44] Prosthetic joint infection (PJI) is an uncommon manifestation, so far described only among elderly immunocompromised hosts in sporadic case reports.[45,46] A recent review of all reported cases from 1977 to 2013 suggested that most cryptococcal OAIs occur among immunocompromised hosts who are not infected with human immunodeficiency virus (HIV), without gender bias, and with mortality correlating with degree of underlying comorbidities.[44] Despite the emergence of *Cryptococcus gattii* as a potent pathogen among immunocompetent hosts in the Pacific Northwest and other areas, OAI caused by this organism has not been reported.

Optimal therapy for cryptococcal OAI in most cases includes a course of induction combination therapy with amphotericin B and flucytosine, followed by up to one year of fluconazole; in the absence of concomitant cryptococcemia, CNS involvement, or multifocal disease, 6 to 12 months of fluconazole alone is recommended in otherwise immunocompetent patients. Depending on the immune status of the patient, long term secondary prophylaxis with fluconazole may be beneficial.[16] The role of surgery is not clear, but it is not necessary in all cases.

THE ENDEMIC DIMORPHIC FUNGI

The endemic dimorphic mycoses, which are caused by *Coccidioides* spp, *Histoplasma capsulatum*, *B dermatitidis*, and *Paracoccidioides brasiliensis*, are geographically circumscribed. By comparison, *Sporothrix schenckii*, which is also a dimorphic pathogen, is distributed worldwide. All are uncommon but well-described causes of human OAI. The incidence of coccidioidomycosis, sporotrichosis, and histoplasmosis may be increasing as the result of an increase in susceptible hosts, such as patients infected with HIV, and of human effects on the environment (*Sporothrix*, *Histoplasma*, and *Coccidioides*).[47–49] As a group, they preferentially cause osteomyelitis of the spine and long bones, and septic arthritis of the knees and wrists. OAIs caused by these organisms are more commonly found in men and are disseminated in 55% of patients. However, each organism differs in its propensity to cause infection of the bone/joint tissues of immunocompromised hosts, and they vary in other important clinical and therapeutic respects. For example, *S schenckii* OAIs are predominantly multifocal, arthrotropic, and seen in immunocompromised hosts, whereas blastomyces and paracoccidioides OAIs are more likely to be isolated, to affect bone, and to be found in otherwise healthy hosts.[2]

C immitis and *Coccidioides posadasii* OAIs generally manifest as vertebral osteomyelitis with or without neurologic or contiguous soft tissue involvement, or as septic arthritis of the knee, wrist, or ankle. Treatment guidelines suggest initial therapy with amphotericin B followed by long-term (3 years or more) treatment with fluconazole or itraconazole. Surgical intervention on coccidioidal spine disease is undertaken for neurologic deficit, persistent instability, intractable pain, or undebrided abscess.[2,17]

H capsulatum, the most frequent endemic mycosis in the United States, is encountered in the Midwest and southeast United States, the Caribbean, and Africa. The epidemiology of this organism, derived from outbreak investigations, suggests common exposures to birds, bats, and construction areas. Its 2 subspecies may differ in clinical presentation: *H capsulatum* var. *capsulatum* (generally isolated in the United States) and var. *duboisii* (generally isolated in Africa). The African subspecies typically causes solitary OAI, and has been reported more commonly among immunocompetent hosts. *H capsulatum* var. *capsulatum* OAI is usually multifocal and seen as part of disseminated disease.[2] Disseminated *Histoplasma* OAIs are noted in patients with immunodeficiencies, including acquired immunodeficiency syndrome, and in the immune reconstitution inflammatory syndrome.[50] Complications of orthopedic surgery caused by this organism are reported.[51] In addition to its rare presentation as a direct cause of OAI, *Histoplasma* can provoke an autoimmune inflammatory arthritis (often in conjunction with erythema nodosum) in the setting of remote primary acute infection.[52] Itraconazole is the antifungal of choice for histoplasma infections, with liposomal amphotericin used for the first 2 to 6 weeks of treatment in severe disease.

Between 25% and 40% of patients with *B dermatitidis* infection, particularly among more immunocompromised hosts, have disseminated infection, including OAI. Blastomyces osteomyelitis usually presents with a solitary lesion and is distinctly more common than septic arthritis. Although mild pulmonary blastomycosis in healthy hosts often resolves without treatment, dissemination can sometimes occur, and treatment is indicated to prevent OAI and other disseminated manifestations. Treatment of *B immitis* OAI generally consists of amphotericin induction followed by oral itraconazole to complete at least 1 year of chemotherapy.

P brasiliensis is a dimorphic fungus endemic to subtropical Latin America, especially Colombia and northern Brazil, for which the development of OAI is rare. Existing cases suggest that, rather than the more common route of airborne infection, paracocci-dioides OAI may also emerge through trauma or direct inoculation, and predominantly among men. Concurrent pulmonary involvement is common. Among the endemic mycoses, only *P brasiliensis* has been reported to rarely present with paradoxic reactions after initiation of antifungal therapy, although such reactions are not reported among cases of OAI.[53] Triazoles, amphotericin B, and cotrimoxazole, uniquely among the endemic fungi, are effective means of treatment.[54]

Talaromyces (Penicillium) marneffei is an emerging southeast Asian endemic fungus with rare osteoarticular manifestations. Host immunity is a critical factor determining risk and manifestations of penicilliosis. Although a large series of 795 patients coinfected with HIV and *P marneffei* from Vietnam failed to identify a single case of OAI,[55] such infections have been reported, and are associated with multifocal lesions and poor outcomes.[2,56–58] Increasing talaromyces infections among immunocompromised hosts not infected with HIV has been noted. Two studies observed an increased incidence of OAI, decreased fungemia, and increased mortality in non–HIV-associated penicilliosis in Thailand and China.[59,60] Triazoles and amphotericin B remain cornerstones of therapy.

Sporotrichosis, a sporadic worldwide mycosis caused by the melaninogenic molds *S schenkii* and *Sporothrix brasiliensis*, typically presents as 1 or more cutaneous lesions near the site of traumatic inoculation on an extremity. Environmental outbreaks from plant sources, such as sphagnum moss,[61] and zoonotic transmissions from toly-peutines, felines, other mammals, and parrots have been reported.[62] Small yeast cells with cigar-shaped budding may be observed in some clinical samples under direct examination, Gram stain, or hematoxylin-eosin; asteroid bodies and Splendore-Hoeppli phenomenon can also be seen. Because the contribution of histopathologic examination to the diagnosis of sporotrichosis may be less than for other endemic mycoses, culture of the biopsy is important for a definitive mycological diagnosis.[2,62] Sporothrix OAI can develop by contiguous or hematogenous spread. Multifocal disease is more common among hosts with impaired immune function. Sporothrical OAI may be underreported.[63] Treatment with 1 year of itraconazole, with or without initial amphotericin B, is recommended.[18] Saturated solution of potassium iodide (SSKI) flucytosine, fluconazole, and voriconazole should not be used for OAI; systemic terbinafine may have activity against *S brasiliensis*.[64–66] Posaconazole and newer azoles may have a role in salvage therapy.[67] The impact of surgery is not well described for *S schenkii* OAI.

Multiple other molds, such as *Scedosporium*, *Fusarium*, and other Mucorales, are very rare causes of fungal OAI. These organisms may cause substantial delays in diagnosis. Because antifungal susceptibility is difficult to predict, combination therapy, often with amphotericin B and voriconazole, is often first-line therapy until susceptibility results are finalized.[68]

PROSTHETIC JOINT INFECTIONS AND OTHER ORTHOPEDIC HARDWARE INFECTIONS

Estimates in the literature are that less than 1% of all PJIs are fungal in cause.[69] Although a wide variety of fungi, including *Aspergillus* spp, *Coccidioides* spp, and *Sporothrix* spp, have been reported, *Candida* spp cause most fungal PJIs, accounting for more than 80% of all cases.[70,71] Concomitant bacterial infection complicated up to one-fifth of these cases.[69] As the population ages and the number of arthroplasties increases, fungal PJIs are likely to become increasingly common. These infections often present indolently, with subacute swelling and pain. Systemic symptoms are unusual, unless the infection has developed in the setting of an overwhelming fungemia. Risk factors for fungal PJI do not seem to be distinct from those for bacterial PJI, although fungal PJIs are reported more commonly following revision arthroplasty.[72]

Successful treatment has been reported in patients undergoing 2-stage exchange, in accordance with the current guidelines from the IDSA,[73] using cement loaded with antifungal agents. The success rate from one series, comprising thirty 2-stage revision procedures in 28 patients, reported a success rate in excess of 90%.[74] However, a contemporary series of similar size reported that less than one-third of patients undergoing resection arthroplasty could be cured with completion of a 2-stage exchange, which is much less than the rate seen in the treatment of bacterial PJIs.[13] Echoing these dismal results is a review of 164 patients from the literature, which found that, of 107 patients who underwent resection arthroplasty and had 2 years of follow-up, only 79 (73.8%) were able to proceed to reimplantation; 28 (26.2%) were unable to be reimplanted.[71] Of the 79 who did complete the second stage, 12 (15%) were not cured and 5 were cured only after addition surgery. Of those who underwent resection arthroplasty, only 57.9% were cured following a 2-stage exchange procedure. Attempts to treat without implant removal have been met with very poor outcomes and this is not recommended, although case reports of successful outcomes with retention of the infected implant have been reported.[75]

The published experience of single-stage revision for fungal PJIs is very limited. The largest series to date, reported from a single center in Germany and comprising 10 patients with candida PJIs, reported a successful outcome in 9, with a mean follow-up period of 7 years.[76] Patients received intravenous antifungal treatment for a mean of 10 days, and were continued on oral treatment for a mean of 5 weeks postoperatively. Further study will be required to determine whether this success can be translated to other centers.

SPECIAL POPULATIONS
Chronic Granulomatous Disease

Chronic granulomatous disease (CGD) is a rare primary immunodeficiency related to mutations in the genes encoding components of the nicotinamide adenine dinucleotide phosphate (NADPH) oxidase system, resulting in impairment of neutrophil microbicidal activity against certain bacterial and fungal pathogens. CGD can present at any time between infancy and late adulthood.[77] In one large series of patients with CGD, *Aspergillus* spp were the most common cause of severe infection, more common than *Staphylococcus aureus*, *Nocardia* spp, *Burkholderia cepacia*, and *Serratia marcescens*, and fungal infections were found to carry a higher risk of mortality than bacterial infections.[78] *Aspergillus* gains entry to the body via the lungs and from there can spread contiguously to the ribs or spine, or spread hematogenously throughout the body to infect a wide array of tissue, including bones and joints.[5,78,79] Because of the defect in neutrophil microbicidal activity, invasive fungal infections may present with few obvious signs or symptoms of inflammation until the process is advanced.

Illicit Intravenous Drug Use

Illicit intravenous drug users are at risk for developing fungal musculoskeletal infections either by hematogenous spread or by direct inoculation. Infections are most often caused by commensal fungi, with C albicans being the most commonly reported cause.[80] Typically, infections develop indolently, primarily within the spine, but can also cause infection at less commonly encountered sites, such as the sacroiliac and sternoclavicular joints. The sites of infection are largely dictated by blood supply and relative levels of vascularity.[81] Intravenous drug users are also at increased risk for fungal infections at other sites, including the heart valves, the eye, and the brain. Increasingly, non-albicans Candida spp have been reported as causing infections in this risk group as well.[82] Intravenous drug users are also at risk for developing osteomyelitis secondary to environmental fungi, such as Aspergillus. Conidia can contaminate the drug supply or the equipment used for injection. This risk increases when drug paraphernalia is shared.[83]

Neonates

Invasive fungal infections in neonates, including bone and joint infections, have become increasingly common over the last several decades.[84] In a prospective registry of more than 6000 very-low-weight infants who had developed late-onset (after 3 days of life) sepsis, C albicans was the third most frequently isolated organism.[85] This finding has been attributed to multiple factors, including the increasing survival rate of preterm infants, the use of parenteral nutrition, intravenous catheters, and broad-spectrum antibiotics.[86] OAI can develop in the setting of acute candidemia, most often with the involvement of other organ systems as well, or can only become apparent weeks to months following the treatment of invasive or disseminated candidiasis.[87]

ANTIFUNGAL PHARMACOLOGY AND OSTEOARTICULAR INFECTIONS

Antifungal therapy for invasive infections is limited to 3 main drugs or classes of drugs: amphotericin B, the triazoles, and the echinocandins. The introduction of amphotericin preceded the other 2 by several decades. It can be very effective when treating invasive fungal infections but its use is limited by dose-limiting nephrotoxicity and infusion-related adverse events, such as chills, myalgias, and joint pain. Newer lipid preparations have decreased the frequency of these side effects. The introduction of fluconazole in 1990 provided clinicians with a much less toxic alterative for susceptible fungi, as well as the ability to treat these infections orally. Newer triazoles, such as voriconazole, posaconazole, and isavuconazole, have expanded the spectrums of activity. Echinocandins were introduced in 2001: caspofungin, the first agent introduced, was followed by anidulafungin and micafungin. This class of parenteral antifungals is well tolerated and effective, especially for osteoarticular candidiasis. The choice of antifungal agent depends mainly on the organism being targeted, because intrinsic resistance to 1 or more classes may exist, and susceptibility patterns may vary even among members of the same genus. A fourth antifungal agent, flucytosine, was originally developed in 1957 as an antimetabolite. It has a limited spectrum of activity and, given the high level of primary and acquired resistance encountered when it is given as monotherapy, it is used only in combination with other antifungal agents. Its use is primarily limited to treatment of cryptococcal infections and some forms of invasive candidal infections. Treatment with flucytosine is further complicated by its significant side effect profile, including hematologic, hepatic, and gastrointestinal toxicity; drug level monitoring can help to limit toxicity.

Antifungal agents may be also often given locally when treating osteomyelitis and PJI, impregnated in polymethyl methacrylate (PMMA) bone cement or calcium sulfate beads.[15] However, although antibiotic-loaded cement is routinely used in the treatment of musculoskeletal and prosthesis-related bacterial infections, and the elution properties of various antibiotics have been well studied, the analogous use of antifungals is much less well understood. Publications on this subject are few, and primarily report on in vitro data.[15,70] Given the heterogeneity of the methodology of these studies, little can conclusively be stated about the elution properties of the antifungals, or their effects on compressive strength, although the available data do suggest that voriconazole may have therapeutic benefit,[88,89] whereas echinocandins may not be suitable for depot delivery.[90,91] Amphotericin has been shown to be stable in cement, although there have been conflicting data as to its ability to elute at therapeutic levels.[92–94] Likewise, the reported clinical experience is also limited; a review of the literature in 2014 found only 7 cases documenting in detail the use of antifungal bone cement in conjunction with clinical outcomes.[95] All 7 were infected with a *Candida* sp and received, in addition to systemic antifungal treatment, either an amphotericin-loaded or fluconazole-loaded spacer or cement beads. Five of the 7 were successfully reimplanted. Elution data were not reported. Adjunctive intraoperative amphotericin B irrigation of infected tissues has also been used to treat candida OAI, but this modality has not been studied in a controlled fashion.[24]

SUMMARY

Fungal bone and joint infections are caused by diverse organisms but are rarely encountered in routine clinical practice. Often, the presentation is subacute, and can be indistinguishable from the more common causes of OAIs. A delay in diagnosis can lead to serious complications. A high index of suspicion is often required to establish the diagnosis and successful treatment often necessitates a complex course of surgical intervention and prolonged use of antifungal therapy. The optimal approach to each patient can vary and depends on the fungus involved, the immune status of the host, the site of infection, and the presence of foreign bodies; close coordination between orthopedists and infectious disease specialists is paramount.

REFERENCES

1. Gamaletsou MN, Walsh TJ, Sipsas NV. Epidemiology of fungal osteomyelitis. Curr Fungal Infect Rep 2014;8(4):262–70.
2. Rammaert B, Gamaletsou MN, Zeller V, et al. Dimorphic fungal osteoarticular infections. Eur J Clin Microbiol Infect Dis 2014;33(12):2131–40.
3. Smith RM, Schaefer MK, Kainer MA, et al. Fungal infections associated with contaminated methylprednisolone injections. N Engl J Med 2013;369(17): 1598–609.
4. Taj-Aldeen SJ, Rammaert B, Gamaletsou M, et al. Osteoarticular infections caused by non-*Aspergillus* filamentous fungi in adult and pediatric patients: a systematic review. Medicine 2015;94(50):e2078.
5. Gamaletsou MN, Rammaert B, Bueno MA, et al. Aspergillus osteomyelitis: epidemiology, clinical manifestations, management, and outcome. J Infect 2014;68(5): 478–93.
6. Gamaletsou MN, Kontoyiannis DP, Sipsas NV, et al. Candida osteomyelitis: analysis of 207 pediatric and adult cases (1970-2011). Clin Infect Dis 2012;55(10): 1338–51.

7. Blyth CC, Gomes L, Sorrell TC, et al. Skull-base osteomyelitis: fungal vs. bacterial infection. Clin Microbiol Infect 2011;17(2):306–11.

8. Zijlstra EE, van de Sande WWJ, Welsh O, et al. Mycetoma: a unique neglected tropical disease. Lancet Infect Dis 2016;16(1):100–12.

9. Tribble DR, Rodriguez CJ. Combat-related invasive fungal wound infections. Curr Fungal Infect Rep 2014;8(4):277–86.

10. Benedict K, Park BJ. Invasive fungal infections after natural disasters. Emerg Infect Dis 2014;20(3):349–55.

11. Fanning S, Mitchell AP. Fungal biofilms. PLoS Pathog 2012;8(4):e1002585.

12. Desai JV, Mitchell AP, Andes DR. Fungal biofilms, drug resistance, and recurrent infection. Cold Spring Harb Perspect Med 2014;4(10). http://dx.doi.org/10.1101/cshperspect.a019729.

13. Azzam K, Parvizi J, Jungkind D, et al. Microbiological, clinical, and surgical features of fungal prosthetic joint infections: a multi-institutional experience. J Bone Joint Surg Am 2009;91(Suppl 6):142–9.

14. Kohli R, Hadley S. Fungal arthritis and osteomyelitis. Infect Dis Clin North Am 2005;19(4):831–51.

15. Bariteau JT, Waryasz GR, McDonnell M, et al. Fungal osteomyelitis and septic arthritis. J Am Acad Orthop Surg 2014;22(6):390–401.

16. Perfect JR, Dismukes WE, Dromer F, et al. Clinical practice guidelines for the management of cryptococcal disease: 2010 update by the Infectious Diseases Society of America. Clin Infect Dis 2010;50(3):291–322.

17. Galgiani JN, Ampel NM, Blair JE, et al. 2016 Infectious Diseases Society of America (IDSA) clinical practice guideline for the treatment of coccidioidomycosis. Clin Infect Dis 2016;63(6):e112–46.

18. Kauffman CA, Bustamante B, Chapman SW, et al, Infectious Diseases Society of America. Clinical practice guidelines for the management of sporotrichosis: 2007 update by the Infectious Diseases Society of America. Clin Infect Dis 2007; 45(10):1255–65.

19. Pappas PG, Kauffman CA, Andes DR, et al. Clinical practice guideline for the management of candidiasis: 2016 update by the Infectious Diseases Society of America. Clin Infect Dis 2016;62(4):e1–50.

20. Patterson TF, Thompson GR, Denning DW, et al. Practice guidelines for the diagnosis and management of aspergillosis: 2016 update by the Infectious Diseases Society of America. Clin Infect Dis 2016;63(4):e1–60.

21. Wheat LJ, Freifeld AG, Kleiman MB, et al. Clinical practice guidelines for the management of patients with histoplasmosis: 2007 update by the Infectious Diseases Society of America. Clin Infect Dis 2007;45(7):807–25.

22. Chapman SW, Dismukes WE, Proia LA, et al. Clinical practice guidelines for the management of blastomycosis: 2008 update by the Infectious Diseases Society of America. Clin Infect Dis 2008;46(12):1801–12.

23. Simitsopoulou M, Peshkova P, Tasina E, et al. Species-specific and drug-specific differences in susceptibility of Candida biofilms to echinocandins: characterization of less common bloodstream isolates. Antimicrob Agents Chemother 2013; 57(6):2562–70.

24. Miller AO, Gamaletsou MN, Henry MW, et al. Successful treatment of Candida osteoarticular infections with limited duration of antifungal therapy and orthopedic surgical intervention. Infect Dis (Lond) 2015;47(3):144–9.

25. Gamaletsou MN, Rammaert B, Bueno MA, et al. Candida arthritis: analysis of 112 pediatric and adult cases. Open Forum Infect Dis 2016;3(1):ofv207.

26. Chatzimoschou A, Katragkou A, Simitsopoulou M, et al. Activities of triazole-echinocandin combinations against *Candida* species in biofilms and as planktonic cells. Antimicrob Agents Chemother 2011;55(5):1968–74.

27. Bouza E, Guinea J, Guembe M. The role of antifungals against *Candida* biofilm in catheter-related candidemia. Antibiotics (Basel, Switzerland) 2014;4(1):1–17.

28. Guembe M, Guinea J, Marcos-Zambrano LJ, et al. Micafungin at physiological serum concentrations shows antifungal activity against *Candida albicans* and Candida parapsilosis biofilms. Antimicrob Agents Chemother 2014;58(9):5581–4.

29. Chowdhary A, Voss A, Meis JF. Multidrug-resistant *Candida auris*: "new kid on the block" in hospital-associated infections? J Hosp Infect 2016;94(3):209–12.

30. Clinical alert to US healthcare facilities - June 2016: Global emergence of invasive infections caused by the multidrug-resistant yeast *Candida auris*. Available at: https://www.cdc.gov/fungal/diseases/candidiasis/candida-auris-alert.html. Accessed September 22, 2016.

31. Chowdhary A, Anil Kumar V, Sharma C, et al. Multidrug-resistant endemic clonal strain of *Candida auris* in India. Eur J Clin Microbiol Infect Dis 2014;33(6):919–26.

32. Cornely OA, Lasso M, Betts R, et al. Caspofungin for the treatment of less common forms of invasive candidiasis. J Antimicrob Chemother 2007;60(2):363–9.

33. Marcos-Zambrano LJ, Escribano P, Bouza E, et al. Comparison of the antifungal activity of micafungin and amphotericin B against *Candida tropicalis* biofilms. J Antimicrob Chemother 2016;71(9):2498–501.

34. Slenker AK, Keith SW, Horn DL. Two hundred and eleven cases of *Candida* osteomyelitis: 17 case reports and a review of the literature. Diagn Microbiol Infect Dis 2012;73(1):89–93.

35. Koehler P, Tacke D, Cornely OA. Aspergillosis of bones and joints - a review from 2002 until today. Mycoses 2014;57(6):323–35.

36. Vinas FC, King PK, Diaz FG. Spinal aspergillus osteomyelitis. Clin Infect Dis 1999; 28(6):1223–9.

37. Sun L, Zhang L, Wang K, et al. Fungal osteomyelitis after arthroscopic anterior cruciate ligament reconstruction: a case report with review of the literature. Knee 2012;19(5):728–31.

38. Cortez KJ, Roilides E, Quiroz-Telles F, et al. Infections caused by *Scedosporium* spp. Clin Microbiol Rev 2008;21(1):157–97.

39. Alastruey-Izquierdo A, Castelli MV, Cuesta I, et al. In vitro activity of antifungals against Zygomycetes. Clin Microbiol Infect 2009;15(Suppl 5):71–6.

40. Kauffman CA, Pappas PG, Patterson TF. Fungal infections associated with contaminated methylprednisolone injections. N Engl J Med 2013;368(26): 2495–500.

41. Fahal AH, Shaheen S, Jones DH. The orthopaedic aspects of mycetoma. Bone Joint J 2014;96-B(3):420–5.

42. Zein HA, Fahal AH, Mahgoub ELS, et al. Predictors of cure, amputation and follow-up dropout among patients with mycetoma seen at the Mycetoma Research Centre, University of Khartoum, Sudan. Trans R Soc Trop Med Hyg 2012;106(11):639–44.

43. Behrman RE, Masci JR, Nicholas P. Cryptococcal skeletal infections: case report and review. Rev Infect Dis 1990;12(2):181–90.

44. Zhou H-X, Lu L, Chu T, et al. Skeletal cryptococcosis from 1977 to 2013. Front Microbiol 2014;5:740.

45. Shah NB, Shoham S, Nayak S. *Cryptococcus neoformans* prosthetic joint infection: case report and review of the literature. Mycopathologia 2015;179(3–4): 275–8.

46. Johannsson B, Callaghan JJ. Prosthetic hip infection due to *Cryptococcus neoformans*: case report. Diagn Microbiol Infect Dis 2009;64(1):76–9.
47. Carlos WG, Rose AS, Wheat LJ, et al. Blastomycosis in Indiana: digging up more cases. Chest 2010;138(6):1377–82.
48. Lortholary O, Denning DW, Dupont B. Endemic mycoses: a treatment update. J Antimicrob Chemother 1999;43(3):321–31.
49. Centers for Disease Control and Prevention (CDC). Increase in reported coccidioidomycosis–United States, 1998-2011. MMWR Morb Mortal Wkly Rep 2013; 62(12):217–21.
50. Marianelli LG, Frassone N, Marino M, et al. Immune reconstitution inflammatory syndrome as histoplasmosis osteomyelitis in South America. AIDS 2014;28(12): 1848–50.
51. Falster L, Marin MB, Gomes JL. Histoplasmosis diagnosed after arthroscopy of the knee: case report. Braz J Infect Dis 2015;19(5):546–8.
52. Rosenthal J, Brandt KD, Wheat LJ, et al. Rheumatologic manifestations of histoplasmosis in the recent Indianapolis epidemic. Arthritis Rheum 1983;26(9): 1065–70.
53. Gryschek RCB, Pereira RM, Kono A, et al. Paradoxical reaction to treatment in 2 patients with severe acute paracoccidioidomycosis: a previously unreported complication and its management with corticosteroids. Clin Infect Dis 2010; 50(10):e56–8.
54. Ferreira MS. Paracoccidioidomycosis. Paediatr Respir Rev 2009;10(4):161–5.
55. Le T, Wolbers M, Chi NH, et al. Epidemiology, seasonality, and predictors of outcome of AIDS-associated *Penicillium marneffei* infection in Ho Chi Minh City, Viet Nam. Clin Infect Dis 2011;52(7):945–52.
56. Louthrenoo W, Thamprasert K, Sirisanthana T. Osteoarticular penicilliosis marneffei. A report of eight cases and review of the literature. Br J Rheumatol 1994; 33(12):1145–50.
57. Chan YF, Woo KC. Penicillium marneffei osteomyelitis. J Bone Joint Surg Br 1990; 72(3):500–3.
58. Pun TS, Fang D. A case of *Penicillium marneffei* osteomyelitis involving the axial skeleton. Hong Kong Med J 2000;6(2):231–3.
59. Kawila R, Chaiwarith R, Supparatpinyo K. Clinical and laboratory characteristics of penicilliosis marneffei among patients with and without HIV infection in northern Thailand: a retrospective study. BMC Infect Dis 2013;13:464.
60. Chan JFW, Lau SKP, Yuen K-Y, et al. *Talaromyces* (*Penicillium*) *marneffei* infection in non-HIV-infected patients. Emerg Microbes Infect 2016;5:e19.
61. Hajjeh R, McDonnell S, Reef S, et al. Outbreak of sporotrichosis among tree nursery workers. J Infect Dis 1997;176(2):499–504.
62. Barros MB, de Almeida Paes R, Schubach AO. *Sporothrix schenckii* and sporotrichosis. Clin Microbiol Rev 2011;24(4):633–54.
63. Howell SJ, Toohey JS. Sporotrichal arthritis in south central Kansas. Clin Orthop Relat Res 1998;346:207–14.
64. Kauffman CA, Pappas PG, McKinsey DS, et al. Treatment of lymphocutaneous and visceral sporotrichosis with fluconazole. Clin Infect Dis 1996;22(1):46–50.
65. Alvarado-Ramírez E, Torres-Rodríguez JM. In vitro susceptibility of *Sporothrix schenckii* to six antifungal agents determined using three different methods. Antimicrob Agents Chemother 2007;51(7):2420–3.
66. Borba-Santos LP, Rodrigues AM, Gagini TB, et al. Susceptibility of *Sporothrix brasiliensis* isolates to amphotericin B, azoles, and terbinafine. Med Mycol 2015; 53(2):178–88.

67. Gutierrez-Galhardo MC, Zancopé-Oliveira RM, Monzón A, et al. Antifungal susceptibility profile in vitro of *Sporothrix schenckii* in two growth phases and by two methods: microdilution and E-test. Mycoses 2010;53(3):227–31.

68. Koehler P, Tacke D, Cornely OA. Bone and joint infections by Mucorales, *Scedosporium, Fusarium* and even rarer fungi. Crit Rev Microbiol 2016;42(1):158–71.

69. Tande AJ, Patel R. Prosthetic joint infection. Clin Microbiol Rev 2014;27(2): 302–45.

70. Jakobs O, Schoof B, Klatte TO, et al. Fungal periprosthetic joint infection in total knee arthroplasty: a systematic review. Orthop Rev (Pavia) 2015;7(1):5623.

71. Kuiper JWP, van den Bekerom MPJ, van der Stappen J, et al. 2-stage revision recommended for treatment of fungal hip and knee prosthetic joint infections. Acta Orthop 2013;84(6):517–23.

72. Parvizi J, Azzam K, Ghanem E, et al. Periprosthetic infection due to resistant staphylococci: serious problems on the horizon. Clin Orthop Relat Res 2009; 467(7):1732–9.

73. Osmon DR, Berbari EF, Berendt AR, et al. Diagnosis and management of prosthetic joint infection: clinical practice guidelines by the Infectious Diseases Society of America. Clin Infect Dis 2013;56(1):e1–25.

74. Hwang BH, Yoon JY, Nam CH, et al. Fungal peri-prosthetic joint infection after primary total knee replacement. J Bone Joint Surg Br 2012;94(5):656–9.

75. Simonian PT, Brause BD, Wickiewicz TL. Candida infection after total knee arthroplasty. Management without resection or amphotericin B. J Arthroplasty 1997; 12(7):825–9.

76. Klatte TO, Kendoff D, Kamath AF, et al. Single-stage revision for fungal periprosthetic joint infection: a single-centre experience. Bone Joint J 2014; 96-B(4):492–6.

77. Goldblatt D, Thrasher AJ. Chronic granulomatous disease. Immunodeficiency review. Clin Exp Immunol 2000;122(1):1–9.

78. Marciano BE, Spalding C, Fitzgerald A, et al. Common severe infections in chronic granulomatous disease. Clin Infect Dis 2015;60(8):1176–83.

79. Bassiri-Jahromi S, Doostkam A. Fungal infection and increased mortality in patients with chronic granulomatous disease. J Mycol Med 2012;22(1):52–7.

80. Bisbe J, Miro JM, Latorre X, et al. Disseminated candidiasis in addicts who use brown heroin: report of 83 cases and review. Clin Infect Dis 1992;15(6):910–23.

81. Levine DP, Brown PD. Infections in injection drug users. In: Bennett JE, Dolin R, Blaser MJ, editors. Mandell, Douglas, and Bennett's principles and practice of infectious diseases. 8th edition. Philadelphia: Elsevier/Saunders; 2015. p. 3475–91.

82. Miller DJ, Mejicano GC. Vertebral osteomyelitis due to *Candida* species: case report and literature review. Clin Infect Dis 2001;33(4):523–30.

83. Trullas J-C, Bisbe J, Miro JM. Aspergillosis in drug addicts. In: Comarú Pasqualotto A, editor. Aspergillosis: from diagnosis to prevention. Dordrecht (The Netherlands): Springer Netherlands; 2010. p. 545–58.

84. Hundalani S, Pammi M. Invasive fungal infections in newborns and current management strategies. Expert Rev Anti Infect Ther 2013;11(7):709–21.

85. Stoll BJ, Hansen N, Fanaroff AA, et al. Late-onset sepsis in very low birth weight neonates: the experience of the NICHD Neonatal Research Network. Pediatrics 2002;110(2 Pt 1):285–91.

86. Saiman L, Ludington E, Pfaller M, et al. Risk factors for candidemia in neonatal intensive care unit patients. The National Epidemiology of Mycosis Survey study group. Pediatr Infect Dis J 2000;19(4):319–24.

87. Harris MC, Pereira GR, Myers MD, et al. Candidal arthritis in infants previously treated for systemic candidiasis during the newborn period: report of three cases. Pediatr Emerg Care 2000;16(4):249–51.
88. Grimsrud C, Raven R, Fothergill AW, et al. The in vitro elution characteristics of antifungal-loaded PMMA bone cement and calcium sulfate bone substitute. Orthopedics 2011;34(8):e378–81.
89. Miller RB, McLaren AC, Pauken C, et al. Voriconazole is delivered from antifungal-loaded bone cement. Clin Orthop Relat Res 2013;471(1):195–200.
90. Sealy PI, Nguyen C, Tucci M, et al. Delivery of antifungal agents using bioactive and nonbioactive bone cements. Ann Pharmacother 2009;43(10):1606–15.
91. Rouse MS, Heijink A, Steckelberg JM, et al. Are anidulafungin or voriconazole released from polymethylmethacrylate in vitro? Clin Orthop Relat Res 2011; 469(5):1466–9.
92. Goss B, Lutton C, Weinrauch P, et al. Elution and mechanical properties of antifungal bone cement. J Arthroplasty 2007;22(6):902–8.
93. Buranapanitkit B, Oungbho K, Ingviya N. The efficacy of hydroxyapatite composite impregnated with amphotericin B. Clin Orthop Relat Res 2005;437:236–41.
94. Kweon C, McLaren AC, Leon C, et al. Amphotericin B delivery from bone cement increases with porosity but strength decreases. Clin Orthop Relat Res 2011; 469(11):3002–7.
95. Goff TAJ, Rambani R, Ng AB. Current concepts in the management of periprosthetic fungal joint infection using antifungal bone cement. Curr Orthop Pract 2014;25(2):169–74.

Mycobacterial Musculoskeletal Infections

John I. Hogan, MD[a], Rocío M. Hurtado, MD, DTM&H[b], Sandra B. Nelson, MD[c],*

KEYWORDS

- *Mycobacterium tuberculosis* • Nontuberculous mycobacteria • Septic arthritis
- Pott's disease • Osteomyelitis • Tenosynovitis

KEY POINTS

- Patients may be predisposed to mycobacterial musculoskeletal infection by virtue of geographic exposure to *Mycobacterium tuberculosis*; cell-mediated immunosuppression, including use of immunomodulatory therapies; or traumatic or postsurgical inoculation of environmental mycobacteria.
- Mycobacteria often cause paucibacillary disease and may be fastidious in their growth characteristics. Diagnosis usually requires culture confirmation but newer molecular technologies offer the potential to identify infecting organisms more rapidly. Sensitivity testing is recommended whenever possible.
- Mycobacterial musculoskeletal infections remain challenging to treat, requiring combination antimycobacterial therapy generally for a minimum of 6 months. Surgical therapy is often required for infection caused by nontuberculous mycobacteria.

INTRODUCTION

Mycobacterial musculoskeletal infections have contributed to significant morbidity for millennia. Researchers have extracted *Mycobacterium tuberculosis* (MTb) DNA from bone lesions of humans who lived more than 9000 years ago.[1] Despite significant advances in modern medicine, these infections remain challenging to manage. Host deficiencies, antibiotic resistance, drug toxicities, limited medication penetration into bone, and complex surgical considerations can all complicate management of these infections. Additional difficulties stem from limited clinical data to guide therapy for patients with severe mycobacterial infections of bones and joints. This article therefore

Disclosures: None of the authors have any relevant disclosures or financial conflicts of interest.
[a] Division of Infectious Diseases, Massachusetts General Hospital, Harvard Medical School, Cox Building, 5th Floor, 55 Fruit Street, Boston, MA 02114, USA; [b] Mycobacterial Diseases Center, Division of Infectious Diseases, Massachusetts General Hospital, Harvard Medical School, Cox Building, 5th Floor, 55 Fruit Street, Boston, MA 02114, USA; [c] Program in Musculoskeletal Infections, Division of Infectious Diseases, Massachusetts General Hospital, Harvard Medical School, Cox Building, 5th Floor, 55 Fruit Street, Boston, MA 02114, USA
* Corresponding author.
E-mail address: sbnelson@mgh.harvard.edu

Infect Dis Clin N Am 31 (2017) 369–382
http://dx.doi.org/10.1016/j.idc.2017.01.007
0891-5520/17/© 2017 Elsevier Inc. All rights reserved.

id.theclinics.com

offers a framework for the approach to musculoskeletal mycobacterial infections, acknowledging that when data are lacking, expert opinion guides much of the management of these infections.

PATHOGENESIS AND HOST RISK FACTORS

Mycobacteria have evolved alongside humans for millennia. Over this period of coevolution, agents of mycobacterial disease have developed a variety of molecular mechanisms that allow them to evade immune detection, avoid destruction within the host, and eventually propagate to effect clinical disease if left unchecked. On initial inhalation, MTb adheres to complement, Fc receptors, and mannose receptors present on the surfaces of macrophages.[2] Like other mycobacteria, the initial stage of infection with this pathogen is characterized by an early transition to the intracellular space. MTb and nontuberculous mycobacteria (NTM) actively infect the same cells that are instrumental in their clearance, and on moving into the intracellular space, they avoid detection by other arms of the immune system. Once inside the macrophage, MTb interferes with the expression of various proteins involved in pH regulation and produces a urease that prevents acidification of the phagosome.[2,3] Other NTM adopt a similar strategy.[4] Mycobacteria, including MTb, are also known to express superoxide dismutase, catalase, and thioredoxin to mitigate the reactive oxygen species produced by phagocytic cells.[5] Even if multiple intracellular mechanisms fail to control the intracellular propagation of mycobacteria, macrophage apoptosis mediated by tumor necrosis factor (TNF)–alpha can limit the propagation and viability of mycobacterial species like MTb.[6] However, virulent strains of MTb may still interfere with macrophage apoptosis, thus enhancing their propagation.[7] After becoming established in the intracellular space, cellular immunity becomes essential in clearing mycobacterial infections. TNF-alpha, interleukin (IL)-12, and interferon (IFN)-gamma help to facilitate control of these primarily intracellular pathogens.

Patients with certain inherited and acquired immunodeficiencies or other medical comorbidities are known to be at higher risk of mycobacterial infection in general (**Box 1**). In addition, use of corticosteroids and other immunomodulatory medications has now become one of the most common factors predisposing to invasive mycobacterial disease. In particular, TNF-alpha modulators confer a significant risk of reactivation of tuberculosis, and a growing number of reports suggest that these agents can also increase the risk of invasive NTM infections.[8–10] Although infliximab and adalimumab seem to confer greater risk than etanercept, all three of these immunomodulators may increase the risk of new or reactivated musculoskeletal infections with acid-fast bacilli (AFB).

RISK FACTORS FOR MUSCULOSKELETAL INVOLVEMENT

In a susceptible host, mycobacterial musculoskeletal infections may occur via several different mechanisms. Tuberculosis generally spreads to osteoarticular sites via the hematogenous route. During primary infection with MTb, bacillemia may occur, although it is usually contained by cell-mediated immunity. When cellular immunity is impaired, bacillemia may lead to seeding of sanctuary sites, including bones and joints. Osteoarticular tuberculosis may manifest during primary infection, although more commonly it represents reactivation of latent bacilli well after an initial bout of primary disease.

Although osteoarticular infection caused by NTM may occur via hematogenous spread in immunodeficient hosts, contiguous and lymphatic spread of NTM infection after percutaneous inoculation provides another route of infection for NTM. NTM are

---

Box 1
Host risk factors for mycobacterial infection

Genetic risks

Mutations that interfere with IFN-gamma production and signaling

Mutations that interfere with IL-12 production and signaling

Mutations that interfere with STAT signaling

MonoMAC syndrome

Chronic granulomatous disease

Acquired immunodeficiencies

Autoantibodies targeting IFN-gamma

Iatrogenic immunosuppression, including corticosteroids and TNF-alpha inhibitors

Medical comorbidities

Human immunodeficiency virus/acquired immunodeficiency syndrome

Malnutrition

Malignancy

Diabetes mellitus

Chronic renal disease

Advanced age

Abbreviations: MonoMAC, monocytopenia and mycobacterial infection; STAT, signal transducer and activator of transcription.

---

ubiquitous within the environment, living commensally within soil and water. Traumatic inoculation via environmental vectors (eg, thorns, wood) or via objects contaminated by soil or water can lead to deposition of the organisms within bone or joint spaces. Animal bites and cutaneous injuries in the setting of saltwater exposure have also facilitated serious musculoskeletal infections with mycobacteria.[11–13] Osteoarticular infection associated with injection drug use, in which injection of nonsterile water leads to hematogenous introduction of NTM, has also been reported.[14]

Iatrogenic infections have also occurred. Corticosteroid injections have been associated with outbreaks of NTM infections in joints,[15] presumably caused by contamination of the solution or lack of sterile procedural preparation. Mycobacterial infections may also occur as a consequence of surgery, including those involving prosthetic joints[16] and osteofixation procedures. Cosmetic procedures may also facilitate the inoculation of mycobacteria into skin and soft tissues[17,18] with contiguous spread to adjacent osteoarticular structures. More recently, medical tourism has become a risk factor for invasive mycobacterial disease.[19] Cosmetic procedures performed abroad using suboptimal infection control practices have contributed to disseminated skin and soft tissue mycobacterial infections that may involve bones and joints by contiguous spread.[20] Contamination of irrigant solutions, injectable medications, and surgical instruments may contribute to infection in cases of lipotourism gone awry.[19]

INCIDENCE OF MUSCULOSKELETAL MYCOBACTERIAL INFECTION

Of more than 250,000 patients with tuberculosis reported in the United States between 1993 and 2006, 19% had extrapulmonary disease, of whom 11.3% (2% of all patients with tuberculosis) had osteoarticular involvement.[21] Infections caused by nontuberculous mycobacteria do not require public health reporting, and therefore their exact incidence is not known. More than 120 different species of NTM can cause human infection; the heterogeneity among this diverse group makes these infections challenging to study systematically. For example, between 1965 and 2003, only 31 cases of vertebral osteomyelitis caused by NTM could be identified in the literature.[22] The exact incidence of osteoarticular NTM infections following certain surgical procedures or occurring in specific immunocompromised populations is also not known but is thought to be low.

CLINICAL MANIFESTATIONS
Tuberculosis

Among cases of osteoarticular tuberculosis, the spine is the most commonly affected site of disease. Up to 50% of osteoarticular cases show vertebral involvement[23–25]; this is followed by native septic arthritis primarily involving large joints such as hips and knees. Small joint septic arthritis and osteomyelitis of the extra-axial skeleton occurs less commonly. Multifocal osteoarticular tuberculosis can also occur.[25] Rarely, tuberculosis may cause prosthetic joint infection.[26] A minority of patients with osteoarticular tuberculosis has concomitant active pulmonary infection. An absence of pulmonary symptoms or radiographic abnormalities should not exclude the diagnosis.

Compared with osteoarticular infections with pyogenic bacteria, infections caused by mycobacteria may present more indolently, evolving over the course of months or even years. Although extracellular pyogenic bacteria effect potent immune activation, mycobacterial infections may elicit a less pronounced initial inflammatory response from the host. In the case of tuberculous septic arthritis, chronic joint effusions and synovitis may be present. When tuberculosis infects prosthetic joints, it typically manifests with pain, swelling, and occasionally drainage from the involved joint. Mycobacterial infections after total knee arthroplasty may become clinically apparent as late as 180 months after arthroplasty.[26] This observation strengthens the hypothesis that MTb infections in prosthetic joints represent latent infection reactivated at the time of surgery. When mycobacterial infections invade deeper osteoarticular structures, a process that initially begins as a synovitis or a periostitis may eventually effect frank erosions of bone. Patients with long-standing infection can eventually develop a significant burden of sequestra and involucra. When liquefied tissue and bone destroyed via caseous necrosis accumulates around a site of infection, a so-called cold abscess may form. Although these collections can contain viable bacilli, they elicit much less inflammation than abscesses containing pyogenic bacteria. When the classic signs of osteoarticular infection are less prominent, other signs and symptoms might raise further suspicion for osteoarticular tuberculosis. Prominent B symptoms, including anorexia, weight loss, fatigue, and night sweats, can all accompany chronic tuberculosis. Regional lymphadenopathy or multiple chronic sinus tracts communicating with bones or joints can also serve as clues.

Spinal osteomyelitis caused by MTb was first described in by Percivall Pott in 1779, and is now commonly referred to as Pott's disease.[27] The anterior portions of the lower thoracic and upper lumbar vertebrae are the most common sites affected by Pott's disease.[28] Although pyogenic bacteria causing vertebral osteomyelitis cause a primary discitis that spreads to adjacent vertebral bodies, MTb classically first infects vertebral bodies. Involvement of the disc space is a later finding, and can be a radiographic clue to the disease. Like other forms of spinal osteomyelitis, Pott's disease may contribute to the development of large paraspinal abscesses. Paraspinal abscesses along the cervical spine may manifest with quadriparesis when compressing the cervical cord or with stridor when compressing the trachea.[23] Pott's disease may be associated with chronic sinus tracts or cold abscesses far removed from the primary site of infection, including the supraclavicular space, the buttocks, and even the popliteal fossa.[2] Despite experiencing frank erosion of bone, patients affected by Pott's disease may lack systemic symptoms, and present only with the insidious onset of gradually worsening back pain. Without treatment, destructive changes contribute to the wedging of adjacent damaged vertebrae, a process that may ultimately culminate in the development of a gibbus deformity. Even after appropriate therapy, deformity may still progress, with many patients experiencing greater than 60° of kyphosis.[29] Neurologic symptoms and true neurologic deficits may occur during the course of disease.[25]

Nontuberculous Mycobacteria

Similar to patients with tuberculosis, patients with musculoskeletal infection caused by NTM may develop subacute to chronic septic arthritis. Vertebral osteomyelitis caused by NTM occurs less commonly than with tuberculosis, and is seen most often in immunocompromised hosts with disseminated infections.[30] NTM also can cause septic tenosynovitis after traumatic inoculation, often in an immunocompetent host. After percutaneous inoculation into soft tissues, NTM may cause a subacute to chronic ulceronodular soft tissue infection that manifests slowly over many months. Although many NTM can cause nodular lymphangitis, the classic syndrome is attributed to *Mycobacterium marinum*, an organism found in saltwater and fishtanks.[31] In chronic soft tissue infection, NTM may extend to involve joints and underlying bone by direct extension. Approximately one-quarter of patients with *M marinum* infection develop tenosynovitis.[32] Although not pathognomonic for tenosynovitis from mycobacterial disease, the presence of so-called rice bodies, white nodules consisting of acidophilic material surrounded by fibrin and collagen embedded within tendon sheaths or bursae, should raise suspicion for the diagnosis.[33] Surgical site infection caused by NTM may manifest with subacute to chronic drainage, multifocal ulceronodular disease, and sinus tracts extending to the deep surgical site.

DIAGNOSIS

Because the treatment of infections caused by mycobacteria require different therapies than those caused by conventional bacterial pathogens, confirming a microbiologic diagnosis is of paramount importance. The diagnosis of mycobacterial musculoskeletal infections may be definite (microbiologically confirmed) or probable (eg, more common in tuberculosis, where there is isolation of mycobacteria at another site, and a concomitant compatible osteoarticular manifestation, with or without compatible histopathology). Attempts at culturing MTb, if successful, provide the additional opportunity for drug-susceptibility testing, which is important given the global distribution of drug resistance. Establishing a microbiologic diagnosis in NTM disease is equally important given the heterogeneity of this group and the differences in susceptibilities to antimicrobials.

Routine laboratory tests are of limited value in diagnosing mycobacterial infection. Abnormal results of noninvasive laboratory assays such as the erythrocyte sedimentation rate and C-reactive protein can increase suspicion for mycobacterial infections of bones and joints. Other noninvasive tests assessing prior exposure to tuberculous antigens, including the purified protein derivative (PPD) test and IFN-gamma release assays (IGRAs), can be helpful, although neither can distinguish between latent and active infection. Further, neither PPD nor IGRA is sensitive or specific enough to make a diagnosis. The absence of positive PPD tests or IGRAs should not exclude a diagnosis of tuberculosis; up to 50% of patients with disseminated tuberculosis have negative PPD tests. However, if either test is positive in a patient presenting with clinical manifestations compatible with osteoarticular tuberculosis, these tests may direct further diagnostics and infection control practices.

Although no single imaging characteristic can definitively differentiate musculoskeletal infections caused by typical pyogenic bacteria from those caused by mycobacteria, radiographic studies can still be important in determining the likelihood of mycobacterial infection. Tuberculous arthritis may be characterized by peripherally located osseous erosions and more gradual narrowing of the joint space than is seen with pyogenic arthrits.[34] Pott's disease has characteristic radiographic features that may help to distinguish it from pyogenic spinal osteomyelitis. These features include multilevel involvement, large paraspinal abscesses, relative sparing of the disc space, and the presence of bone fragments.[34] Angular kyphosis is a later finding. Although plain films may be sufficient to distinguish between pyogenic and tuberculous spinal osteomyelitis in later disease, MRI offers greater sensitivity in early disease and improved resolution of soft tissue findings. MRI may identify rice bodies, providing another clue to mycobacterial infection. Although no single radiographic finding is pathognomonic for mycobacterial infection, MRI and other imaging modalities can be used to characterize the extent of disease and identify structures most heavily affected by infection to guide more invasive diagnostics and source control.

Once suggested by history, laboratory tests, and imaging, more invasive diagnostics are generally required to secure the diagnosis of musculoskeletal mycobacterial infection. Synovial fluid aspiration is the first test of choice for the diagnosis of septic arthritis, although it may not yield a firm diagnosis. Compared with conventional pyogenic arthritis, joints infected with mycobacteria typically yield lower synovial cell counts. One review of 40 patients identified an average leukocyte count of 18,062 cells/μL in patients with tuberculosis arthritis compared with 31,250 cells/μL in joints infected with NTM,[30] both of which are lower than is typically seen in bacterial septic arthritis. In this study, 14% of tuberculous effusions yielded AFB on staining, whereas 25% of the NTM effusions stained positive for AFB.[30] The authors recommend that AFB staining be performed on synovial fluid samples. Although the growth of MTb in culture is optimal to confirm the diagnosis, synovial fluid culture may not yield a diagnosis. One review of 31 cases of large joint effusions caused by tuberculosis showed that cultures of joint aspirates yielded a positive result in 61% of these cases.[30] Similar to cultures of peritoneal and pleural fluid, synovial fluid culture has a lower sensitivity than tissue culture, a finding that underscores the importance of obtaining tissue samples to increase the likelihood of making a diagnosis.

Percutaneous or operative biopsy of synovium, bone, cartilage, or adjacent abscess material offers the best chance of securing a diagnosis. Histology performed on infected tissue obtained from an immunocompetent host often detects either necrotizing or non-necrotizing granulomas, and occasionally yields AFB on staining. However, even the microscopic examination of grossly infected tissue may fail to identify the offending pathogen,[35] and culture of infected tissue remains the gold standard for diagnosis. Because multiple sites may be involved in patients with disseminated tuberculosis and NTM, clinicians may also consider sampling other sources for mycobacteria, including blood, sputum, urine, and lymph nodes, in an attempt to isolate a mycobacterial pathogen.

Although the morphologic appearance and growth rate of AFB in culture can provide early clues to the identity of the infecting species, final results using conventional methods take longer to provide species-level identification. Rapidly growing NTM may be identified in days, although the isolation and identification of MTb and slow-growing NTM may take up to 8 weeks or longer. Direct nucleic acid amplification may provide more rapid species-level identification and evidence of anti-microbial resistance genes once an organism has grown in the laboratory, although culture remains imperative for sensitivity testing to fully inform antibiotic selections. One group showed that polymerase chain reaction (PCR) correctly identified MTb in soft tissue specimens obtained from 4 joints infected with this pathogen.[35] Another group reported that, using tissue samples from 19 patients with culture-confirmed Pott's disease, PCR had a sensitivity of 94.7% and a specificity of 83.3%.[36] In cases in which mycobacterial infection is suspected but culture results are negative, PCR may be able to identify a pathogen, although without the important benefit of suscep-tibility results. However, few data are available on the sensitivity and specificity of PCR in the diagnosis of culture-negative tuberculosis, or in osteoarticular infections caused by NTM. Molecular tests may still be useful in the detection of fastidious mycobacteria such as *Mycobacterium genavense*, particularly when conventional mycobacterial culture fails to identify an organism. Given the ubiquity of environmental mycobacteria, and because PCR cannot distinguish between infecting and contaminating organ-isms, care to exclude specimen contamination before testing is imperative. Molecular probes assessing for the presence of genes that confer resistance to specific antibi-otics have the potential to rapidly identify resistant isolates. The GeneXpert nucleic acid amplification assay for rifampin (RIF) resistance in MTb is one of the most commonly used assays of this kind. Although the use of such tests may prove useful, the operating characteristics of these molecular assays have not been thoroughly vali-dated for use in osteoarticular infections.

THERAPY FOR MYCOBACTERIAL MUSCULOSKELETAL INFECTIONS
General Approaches

Once the diagnosis of musculoskeletal mycobacterial infections is suspected or confirmed, medical management should be planned, and surgical management may need to be considered. Although virtually all musculoskeletal mycobacterial infections require medical therapy, some can be managed with close monitoring but without the need for surgery. Care teams consisting of infectious disease specialists, orthopedic surgeons, rheumatologists, and radiologists may work together to determine optimal therapeutic approaches. Because of the potential toxicity of mycobacterial therapy and the potential for drug interactions, a careful understanding of comorbidities and other medications is necessary. For patients receiving immunomodulatory therapy, strong consideration should be given to stopping immunosuppressive medications, particularly TNF-alpha inhibitors, or substituting with less immunosuppressive alterna-tives. The diagnosis of tuberculosis may also confer important public health and infec-tion control considerations.

Mycobacterium tuberculosis

The initial management of osteoarticular tuberculosis consists of early and effective antitubercular therapy, assessment of complications that may merit additional inter-vention, and repeated assessments of clinical response over time to assist in determi-nation of the ultimate length of therapy. Initial medical therapy for drug-susceptible tuberculosis consists of a combination of drugs including rifampin (RIF), isoniazid (iso-nicotinylhydrazine [INH]), pyrazinamide (PZA), and ethambutol (EMB) administered over a period of 2 months[37] (**Table 1**). Of these agents, INH and RIF possess the

Table 1
Initial antibiotic regimens frequently used for common osteoarticular mycobacterial infections[a]

Species	Drug Regimen
MTb	Rifampin plus isoniazid plus pyrazinamide plus EMB
Mycobacterium avium complex[b]	Rifampin plus (azithromycin or clarithromycin) plus EMB
Mycobacterium kansasii	Rifampin plus isoniazid[c] plus EMB
Mycobacterium marinum	Rifampin plus EMB plus (azithromycin or clarithromycin)
Mycobacterium abscessus	(Clarithromycin or azithromycin)[d] plus amikacin plus (cefoxitin or imipenem)
Mycobacterium fortuitum[e]	Amikacin plus trimethoprim/sulfamethoxazole plus quinolone
Mycobacterium chelonae	(Clarithromycin or azithromycin) plus tobramycin plus imipenem

[a] Antimicrobial sensitivities and host factors ultimately dictate the choice of therapy. This table outlines some of the antimicrobial regimens frequently used for sensitive isolates (or as empiric therapy if treatment is started before availability of drug-susceptibility testing). Additional information is available in published treatment guidelines.[8,37] Please note that only a few laboratories screen for inducible macrolide resistance (caused by the *erm* gene) in rapid growers; this may therefore affect the accuracy of macrolide susceptibility results.

[b] If the pathogen is sensitive to amikacin, providers may consider adding this agent to the initial regimen to address severe infections.

[c] Azithromycin and clarithromycin are also active against most isolates. In certain settings, providers may consider substituting azithromycin or clarithromycin for isoniazid. There is controversy regarding the clinical significance of the low-level isoniazid resistance that is sometimes noted in susceptibility testing. All isolates must be tested for rifamycin resistance. Rifamycin sensitivity correlates well with clinical outcomes.

[d] *M abscessus* isolates other than subspecies *massiliense* are frequently resistant to macrolides (inducible resistance). If the isolate is known to be resistant to clarithromycin/azithromycin, providers may instead use tigecycline.

[e] Inducible macrolide resistance is common, and therefore macrolides are often not active agents for this infection.

most potent early antibacillary effect, and should be included in the regimen whenever possible.[23] Antimycobacterial agents achieve sufficient levels within nonsclerotic bone to achieve bactericidal activity against MTb.[38] After the induction period, patients with drug-susceptible disease should continue for an additional 4 to 10 more months of therapy, ideally with INH and RIF depending on clinical and radiographic evolution. During this continuation phase of therapy, RIF becomes especially important in eradicating quiescent bacilli.[23] In patients who cannot tolerate or have isolates resistant to 1 or more of the antimicrobials listed earlier, guidelines are available through the American Thoracic Society (ATS), the Centers for Disease Control and Prevention (CDC), and the Infectious Diseases Society of America (IDSA).[37,39] Expert consultation should guide therapeutic decisions. Some data suggest that therapeutic drug monitoring may optimize clinical outcomes.[40] The authors recommend that, whenever possible, physicians should monitor drug levels to ensure that they are within the therapeutic range for infections in sanctuary sites such as bone, although the direct impact on outcomes remains unknown.

Although the standard antibiotic regimen used to treat susceptible pulmonary tuberculosis is widely accepted, the optimal duration of medical therapy for patients presenting with tuberculous infections of bones and joints is less well defined. Most of the knowledge comes from studies on spinal tuberculosis. One of the first studies to address this question came from the Tenth Report of the Medical Research Council Working Party on Tuberculosis of the Spine.[41] In this 1986 study, 51 patients with Pott's disease underwent excision of diseased bone with placement of bone graft (Hong Kong procedure) followed by 6 months of INH/RIF/streptomycin or the same treatment followed by 3 additional months of INH/RIF. All but 1 of the patients had a favorable clinical outcome at 3 years, suggesting that 9 months of therapy may offer little benefit compared with 6 months. Another trial randomized 256 patients to 1 of 4 treatment groups: 6 months of INH/RIF, 9 months of INH/RIF, 9 months of INH plus either EMB or para-aminosalicylic acid (PAS), or 18 months of INH plus either EMB or PAS.[42] Overall, only 8% of the patients experienced an adverse clinical outcome at 3 years, although the rate was 19% for those receiving 9 months of INH plus either EMB or PAS. This trial suggests that a 6-month course of INH/RIF is adequate for most cases of Pott's disease, although if an alternative regimen (INH plus EMB or PAS) is needed the course should be extended to 18 months. In addition, a 5-year study randomized 451 ambulatory patients with Pott's disease to 6 months of INH/RIF, 9 months of INH/RIF, surgical intervention followed by 6 months of INH/RIF, 9 months of INH plus either EMB or PAS, or 18 months of INH plus either EMB or PAS.[43] After 5 years, only the group that received 9 months of INH plus either EMB or PAS experienced a higher rate of adverse outcomes. These results and others prompt us to treat patients with tuberculous musculoskeletal infections with a minimum of 6 months of potent therapy, preferably containing a backbone of INH/RIF. Therapy may be extended to 9 to 12 months in patients who initially present with a significant burden of disease or when the net state of immunosuppression is high. Treatment courses of 18 months or longer should be considered when INH/RIF cannot be used.

Many cases of spinal tuberculosis can be managed without operative debridement, although the data to guide decisions around surgery are more limited and are based largely on expert opinion. In ambulatory patients, resection of infected bone and placement of bone graft confers no major advantage over medical therapy alone.[41,43] ATS/CDC/IDSA guidelines suggest surgery should be considered for patients with Pott's disease who have significant neurologic deficits related to cord compression, an unstable spine predisposing to cord injury, and those who do not respond to medical therapy.[37] Although surgery is not always necessary for cure, the role of stabilizing surgery for Pott's disease to decrease long-term spinal deformity remains controversial. Some experts also favor operative intervention in patients with very large abscesses or those with a significant burden of devitalized or sclerotic bone in the spine.[38,44,45]

As in Pott's disease, extra-axial tuberculosis can often be managed with medical therapy alone.[45] Large abscesses and significant devitalized bone should be considered for surgery. In cases of septic arthritis failing medical therapy, debridement may improve functional outcomes. Patients with substantial joint destruction characterized by significant loss of joint space and those with fibrous ankylosis with significant loss of function or chronic pain may also benefit from operative management. Physicians may consider excisional arthroplasty or arthrodesis to improve mobility and minimize chronic discomfort.[45] Optimally, total joint arthroplasty after tuberculosis arthritis should be deferred until patients show no evidence of recurrent disease after completion of therapy given the potential for reactivation disease after arthroplasty.[46] The duration of time necessary to exonerate the potential for reactivation is not known; one author recommends several years off antibiotics before arthroplasty and an additional 3 to 5 months of therapy after arthroplasty to prevent reactivation.[45] Although total joint arthroplasty during the phase of active medical treatment of tuberculosis is not preferred, in some settings it may be unavoidable, and in these cases arthroplasty followed by long-term antimycobacterial therapy may be used with some success.[47]

The surgical management of prosthetic joint infection related to MTb is controversial. The authors recommend that large effusions be drained, and that devitalized tissue and purulence be debrided. Because tuberculosis does not form biofilms to the extent that *Staphylococcus* and other typical bacterial species do, hardware may be successfully retained in many cases of MTb prosthetic joint infection.[25] Incision and drainage with liner exchange may be sufficient for many cases of prosthetic joint infection caused by MTb. Complicated infections characterized by hardware loosening, exposed hardware, or the formation of a significant burden of involucra or sequestra should prompt providers to consider removing the prosthesis. It is not known whether a 2-stage hardware management strategy offers any benefit compared with a 1-stage exchange in such cases. Expert opinion guides much of the surgical management of complicated prosthetic joint infections related to MTb.

Nontuberculous Mycobacteria

Much of what is known about the management of osteoarticular infections caused by NTM is either derived from case reports and case series or extrapolated from the tuberculosis literature. The ATS and IDSA have published useful general guidelines discussing therapy for these infections.[8] A minimum of 6 months of multidrug therapy guided by antibiotic sensitivities is usually required for treatment of NTM musculoskeletal infection. However, the optimal length of therapy is not known. Factors including disease burden, virulence of the infecting species, efficacy of available antimycobacterial drugs, degree of host immunosuppression, completeness of surgical debridement (when undertaken), and clinical response affect decision making regarding the duration of therapy. Treatment durations of 12 months or longer may be warranted for severe infections. In the case of more resistant pathogens, such as *Mycobacterium abscessus*, physicians may need to use combination intravenous antibiotics over a prolonged period, and drug toxicity may also contribute to decisions about therapy duration.

In contrast with tuberculosis, osteoarticular infections caused by NTM often require combined medical and surgical management. NTM are intrinsically more resistant to antimycobacterial therapy compared with MTb, and thorough surgical debridement is often necessary for clinical cure. Even with thorough debridement and appropriate medical therapy, infection may recur and necessitate repeated debridement for infection control. In the setting of prosthetic material, successful eradication of NTM infection is unlikely, and hardware removal is recommended to facilitate cure whenever possible. Although there are few case reports describing patients with prosthetic joint infection caused by NTM species successfully treated with hardware retention,[48] the risk of recurrent infection is unknown but is thought to be high. Limited choices for safe long-term suppression of many NTM in the setting of retained hardware further limit this option. Clinicians may consider hardware retention with long-term suppression for less aggressive NTM infections that are sensitive to safe oral antibiotics, although the risk of relapse is unknown and few data exist to guide these decisions.

If prosthetic material is removed, the authors recommend the use of antibiotic-eluting polymethyl methacrylate cement for local delivery of effective antimycobacterial therapy. Many agents active against NTM are thermostable and can be incorporated into cement, including aminoglycosides, some cephalosporins, macrolides, carbapenems, and quinolones.[49] However, the recommended antibiotic doses for cement are based on minimal inhibitory concentrations (MICs) against conventional pyogenic bacteria. As these drugs require higher MICs to target mycobacteria, higher antibiotic doses in cement may be necessary to achieve the desired local tissue concentration. However, the higher antibiotic doses may be offset by loss of stability of the cement, which can lead to fracturing, and the risk of systemic antimicrobial toxicity, particularly with amino-glycosides.[50] Involvement of infectious diseases pharmacists can be particularly useful as antimicrobial selection and dosing for spacers is considered.[51]

SUMMARY

Although less common as causes of musculoskeletal infection than pyogenic bacteria, mycobacterial musculoskeletal infections remain important causes of morbidity worldwide. Although tuberculous arthritis and osteomyelitis have been recognized for millennia, infections caused by NTM are being identified more often, likely because of both a more susceptible host population and improvements in diagnostic capabilities. Infections caused by mycobacteria remain challenging to diagnose, because of the paucibacillary nature of musculoskeletal infection and fastidious growth character-istics. Despite improvements in molecular diagnostic approaches to mycobacterial infection, culture-based diagnosis remains critical for susceptibility testing, which is paramount to guide treatment decisions. The role of surgery in tuberculous arthritis and osteomyelitis is controversial, but many patients with drug-susceptible disease can be cured without surgery. Because of intrinsically greater resistance among NTM, surgical management is usually required for cure. Although modern surgical and medical therapies afford cure in most cases, substantial long-term morbidity may still result. The limited understanding of these complicated infections under-scores the need for higher quality data in the future to guide patient care.

REFERENCES

1. Hershkovitz I, Donoghue HD, Minnikin DE, et al. Detection and molecular charac-terization of 9000-year-old *Mycobacterium tuberculosis* from a Neolithic settle-ment in the eastern Mediterranean. PLoS One 2008;3(10):e3426.
2. Bennett JE, Dolin R, Blaser MJ, et al. Mandell, Douglas, and Bennett's principles and practice of infectious diseases. 8th edition. Philadelphia: Elsevier/Saunders; 2015.
3. Glickman MS, Jacobs WR Jr. Microbial pathogenesis of *Mycobacterium tubercu-losis*: dawn of a discipline. Cell 2001;104(4):477–85.
4. Sturgillkoszycki S, Schlesinger PH, Chakraborty P, et al. Lack of acidification in *Mycobacterium* phagosomes produced by exclusion of the vesicular proton-ATPase. Science 1994;263(5147):678–81.
5. Edwards KM, Cynamon MH, Voladri RK, et al. Iron-cofactored superoxide dismut-ase inhibits host responses to *Mycobacterium tuberculosis*. Am J Respir Crit Care Med 2001;164:2213–9.
6. Oddo M, Renno T, Attinger A, et al. Fas ligand-induced apoptosis of infected hu-man macrophages reduces the viability of intracellular *Mycobacterium tubercu-losis*. J Immunol 1998;160(11):5448–54.
7. Keane J, Remold HG, Kornfeld H. Virulent *Mycobacterium tuberculosis* strains evade apoptosis of infected alveolar macrophages. J Immunol 2000;164(4): 2016–20.
8. Griffith DE, Aksamit T, Brown-Elliott BA, et al. An official ATS/IDSA statement: diagnosis, treatment, and prevention of nontuberculous mycobacterial diseases. Am J Respir Crit Care Med 2007;175(4):367–416.

9. Keane J, Gershon S, Wise RP, et al. Tuberculosis associated with infliximab, a tumor necrosis factor alpha-neutralizing agent. N Engl J Med 2001;345:1098–104.

10. Keane J. Tumor necrosis factor blockers and reactivation of latent tuberculosis. Clin Infect Dis 2004;39:300–2.

11. Hofer M, Hirschel B, Kirschner P, et al. Brief report: disseminated osteomyelitis from *Mycobacterium ulcerans* after a snakebite. N Engl J Med 1993;328(14): 1007–9.

12. Clark RB, Spector H, Friedman DM, et al. Osteomyelitis and synovitis produced by *Mycobacterium marinum* in a fisherman. J Clin Microbiol 1990;28(11):2570–2.

13. Earl T. A chigger bite activates a dormant infection in an outdoorsman. J Am Acad Physician Assist 2010;23(12):1–3.

14. Longardner K, Allen A, Ramgopal M. Spinal osteomyelitis due to *Mycobacterium fortuitum* in a former intravenous drug user. BMJ Case Rep 2013;2013.

15. Jung SY, Kim BG, Kwon D, et al. An outbreak of joint and cutaneous infections caused by non-tuberculous mycobacteria after corticosteroid injection. Int J Infect Dis 2015;36:62–9.

16. Cheung IK, Wilson A. Arthroplasty tourism. Med J Aust 2007;187(11):666–7.

17. Winthrop KL, Abrams M, Yakrus M, et al. An outbreak of mycobacterial furunculosis associated with footbaths at a nail salon. N Engl J Med 2002;326(18): 1366–71.

18. Difonzo EM, Campanile GL, Vanzi L, et al. Mesotherapy and cutaneous *Mycobacterium fortuitum* infection. Int J Dermatol 2009;48(6):645–7.

19. Furuya EY, Paez A, Srinivasan A, et al. Outbreak of *Mycobacterium abscessus* wound infections among "lipotourists" from the United States who underwent abdominoplasty in the Dominican Republic. Clin Infect Dis 2007;46(8):1181–8.

20. Ruegg E, Cheretakis A, Modarressi A, et al. Multisite infection with *Mycobacterium abscessus* after replacement of breast implants and gluteal lipofilling. Case Rep Infect Dis 2015;2015:1–6.

21. Peto HM, Pratt RH, Harrington TA, et al. Epidemiology of extrapulmonary tuberculosis in the United States, 1993–2006. Clin Infect Dis 2009;49(9):1350–7.

22. Petitjean G, Fluckiger U, Schären S, et al. Vertebral osteomyelitis caused by non-tuberculous mycobacteria. Clin Microbiol Infect 2004;10(11):951–3.

23. Koopman WJ, Moreland LW. Arthritis and allied conditions. 15th edition. Philadelphia: Lippincott Williams & Wilkins; 2005.

24. Rasouli MR, Mirkoohi M, Vaccaro AR, et al. Spinal tuberculosis: diagnosis and management. Asian Spine J 2012;6(4):294–308.

25. Johansen IS, Nielsen SL, Hove M, et al. Characteristics and clinical outcome of bone and joint tuberculosis from 1994 to 2011: a retrospective register-based study in Denmark. Clin Infect Dis 2015;61(4):554–62.

26. Kim SJ, Kim JH. Late onset *Mycobacterium tuberculosis* infection after total knee arthroplasty: a systematic review and pooled analysis. Scand J Infect Dis 2013; 45:907–14.

27. Pott P. The chirurgical works of Percivall Pott, F.R.S., surgeon to St. Bartholomew's Hospital, a new edition, with his last corrections. 1808. Clin Orthop Relat Res 2002;(398):4–10.

28. Gouliamos AD, Kehagias DT, Lahanis S, et al. MRI findings in tuberculous vertebral osteomyelitis: a pictorial review. Eur Radiol 2001;11(4):575–9.

29. Rajasekaran S. The problem of deformity in spinal tuberculosis. Clin Orthop Relat Res 2002;398:85–92.

30. Shu CC, Wang JY, Yu CJ, et al. Mycobacterial arthritis of large joints. Ann Rhem Dis 2009;68(9):1504–5.

31. Lam A, Toma W, Schlesinger N. *Mycobacterium marinum* arthritis mimicking rheumatoid arthritis. J Rheumatol 2006;33(4):817–9.

32. Aubry A, Chosidow O, Caumes E, et al. Sixty-three cases of *Mycobacterium marinum* infection: clinical features, treatment, and antibiotic susceptibility of causative isolates. Arch Intern Med 2002;162(15):1746–52.

33. Lee EY, Rubin DA, Brown DM. Recurrent *Mycobacterium marinum* tenosynovitis of the wrist mimicking extraarticular synovial chondromatosis on MR images. Skeletal Radiol 2004;33(7):405–8.

34. Griffith JF, Kumta SM, Leung PC, et al. Imaging of musculoskeletal tuberculosis: a new look at an old disease. Clin Orthop Relat Res 2002;398:32–9.

35. Dionisios V, Kazakos C, Tilkeridis C, et al. Polymerase chain reaction for the detection of *Mycobacterium tuberculosis* in synovial fluid, tissue samples, bone marrow aspirate and peripheral blood. Acta Orthop Belg 2003;69(5):366–9.

36. Berk RH, Yazici M, Atabey N, et al. Detection of *Mycobacterium tuberculosis* in formaldehyde solution-fixed, paraffin-embedded tissue by polymerase chain reaction in Pott's disease. Spine 1996;21(17):1991–5.

37. Nahid P, Dorman SE, Alipanah N, et al. Official American Thoracic Society/Centers for Disease Control and Prevention/Infectious Diseases Society of America clinical practice guidelines: treatment of drug-susceptible tuberculosis. Clin Infect Dis 2016;63(7):e147–95.

38. Ge Z, Wang Z, Wei M. Measurement of the concentration of three antituberculosis drugs in the focus of spinal tuberculosis. Eur Spine J 2008;17(11):1482–7.

39. Treatment of tuberculosis. Centers for Disease Control and Prevention Website. 2003. Available at: http://www.cdc.gov/mmwr/preview/mmwrhtml/rr5211a1.htm. Accessed September 1, 2016.

40. Alsultan A, Peloquin CA. Therapeutic drug monitoring in the treatment of tuberculosis: an update. Drugs 2014;74(8):839–54.

41. A controlled trial of six-month and nine-month regimens of chemotherapy in patients undergoing radical surgery for tuberculosis of the spine in Hong Kong. Tenth report of the Medical Research Council Working Party on Tuberculosis of the Spine. Tubercle 1986;67(4):243–59.

42. Controlled trial of short-course regimens of chemotherapy in the ambulatory treatment of spinal tuberculosis. Results at three years of a study in Korea. Twelfth report of the Medical Research Council Working Party on Tuberculosis of the Spine. J Bone Joint Surg Br 1993;75(2):240–8.

43. Five-year assessment of controlled trials of short-course chemotherapy regimens of 6, 9 or 18 months' duration for spinal tuberculosis in patients ambulatory from the start or undergoing radical surgery. Fourteenth report of the Medical Research Council Working Party on Tuberculosis of the Spine. Int Orthop 1999;23(2):73–81.

44. Liu P, Zhu Q, Jiang J. Distribution of three antituberculous drugs and their metabolites in different parts of pathological vertebrae with spinal tuberculosis. Spine 2011;36(20):E1290–5.

45. Tuli SM. General principles of osteoarticular tuberculosis. Clin Orthop Relat Res 2002;389:11–9.

46. Berbari EF, Hanssen AD, Duffy MC, et al. Prosthetic joint infection due to *Mycobacterium tuberculosis*: a case series and review of the literature. Am J Orthop 1998;27(3):219–27.

47. Neogi DS, Yadav CS, Ashok Kumar, et al. Total hip arthroplasty in patients with active tuberculosis of the hip with advanced arthritis. Clin Orthop Relat Res 2010;468:605–12.

48. Eid AJ, Berbari EF, Sia IG, et al. Prosthetic joint infection due to rapidly growing mycobacteria: report of 8 cases and review of the literature. Clin Infect Dis 2007; 45(6):687–94.
49. Citak M, Argenson JN, Masri B, et al. Spacers. J Arthroplasty 2014;29(2 Suppl): 93–9.
50. Prink M, Eckoff DG. *Mycobacterium chelonae* infection following a total knee arthroplasty. J Arthroplasty 1996;11(1):115–6.
51. Curtis JM, Sternhagen V, Batts D. Acute renal failure after placement of tobramycin-impregnated bone cement in an infected total knee arthroplasty. Pharmacotherapy 2005;25(6):876–80.

Index

Note: Page numbers of article titles are in **boldface** type.

A

Abscess(es)
    psoas muscle, 289–293
    pyomyositis
        radiologic approach to, 303–305
Acute hematogenous osteomyelitis
    in children
        clinical presentation of, 331–332
Acute phase reactants
    in reactive arthritis diagnosis, 270
Amputation
    in PJI management, 246
Anemia
    infection in orthopedic prosthetic surgery related to, 255
Animal bites
    septic arthritis related to, 209
Antibiotic(s)
    in infection prevention in open fractures, 341–345
        choice of, 342–343
        duration of, 344
        local therapy, 344–345
        role of, 341
        timing of, 341–342
        wound cultures and, 343–344
    in orthopedic prosthetic surgery infection prevention, 256–257
    in PJI management, 246–247
    for septic arthritis of native joints, 212–213
Antibiotic-impregnated bone cement
    in orthopedic prosthetic surgery infection prevention, 257
Antibiotic-laden implants
    in orthopedic prosthetic surgery infection prevention, 257
Arthritis
    of native joints
        gonococcal, 207–208
        meningococcal, 208
    reactive, **265–277** See also Reactive arthritis
    rheumatoid
        infection in orthopedic prosthetic surgery related to, 255–256
    septic See Septic arthritis

Moving?

Make sure your subscription moves with you!

To notify us of your new address, find your **Clinics Account Number** (located on your mailing label above your name), and contact customer service at:

Email: journalscustomerservice-usa@elsevier.com

800-654-2452 (subscribers in the U.S. & Canada)
314-447-8871 (subscribers outside of the U.S. & Canada)

Fax number: 314-447-8029

Elsevier Health Sciences Division
Subscription Customer Service
3251 Riverport Lane
Maryland Heights, MO 63043

*To ensure uninterrupted delivery of your subscription, please notify us at least 4 weeks in advance of move.

Printed and bound by CPI Group (UK) Ltd, Croydon, CR0 4YY

08/05/2025

01864699-0011